MW00453216

The 30-Minute Low-FODMAP Cookbook

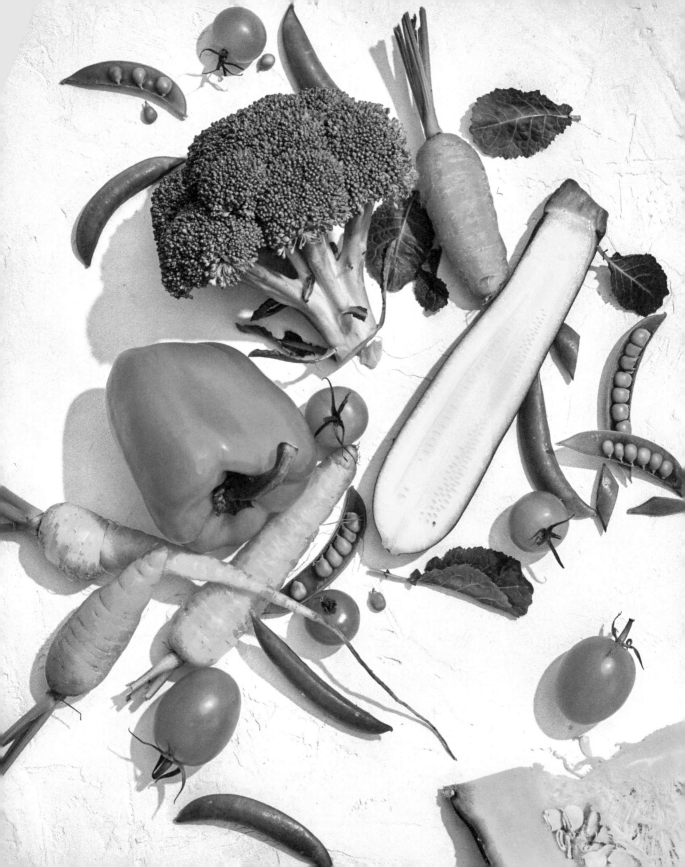

THE 30-MINUTE LOW-FODMAP COOKBOOK

101 Delicious Recipes to Soothe IBS and Other Digestive Disorders

Colleen Francioli, CNC
Photography by Biz Jones

ROCKRIDGE
PRESS

Copyright © 2019 by Rockridge Press, Emeryville, California

No part of this publication may be reproduced, stored in a retrieval system, or transmitted in any form or by any means, electronic, mechanical, photocopying, recording, scanning, or otherwise, except as permitted under Sections 107 or 108 of the 1976 United States Copyright Act, without the prior written permission of the Publisher. Requests to the Publisher for permission should be addressed to the Permissions Department, Rockridge Press, 6005 Shellmound Street, Suite 175, Emeryville CA 94608.

Limit of Liability/Disclaimer of Warranty: The Publisher and the author make no representations or warranties with respect to the accuracy or completeness of the contents of this work and specifically disclaim all warranties, including without limitation warranties of fitness for a particular purpose. No warranty may be created or extended by sales or promotional materials. The advice and strategies contained herein may not be suitable for every situation. This work is sold with the understanding that the Publisher is not engaged in rendering medical, legal, or other professional advice or services. If professional assistance is required, the services of a competent professional person should be sought. Neither the Publisher nor the author shall be liable for damages arising herefrom. The fact that an individual, organization, or website is referred to in this work as a citation and/or potential source of further information does not mean that the author or the Publisher endorses the information the individual, organization, or website may provide or recommendations they/it may make. Further, readers should be aware that websites listed in this work may have changed or disappeared between when this work was written and when it is read.

For general information on our other products and services or to obtain technical support, please contact our Customer Care Department within the United States at (866) 744-2665, or outside the United States at (510) 253-0500.

Rockridge Press publishes its books in a variety of electronic and print formats. Some content that appears in print may not be available in electronic books, and vice versa.

TRADEMARKS: Rockridge Press and the Rockridge Press logo are trademarks or registered trademarks of Callisto Media Inc. and/or its affiliates, in the United States and other countries, and may not be used without written permission. All other trademarks are the property of their respective owners. Rockridge Press is not associated with any product or vendor mentioned in this book.

Interior and Cover Designer: Erik Jacobsen
Art Producer: Hillary Frileck
Editor: Sean Newcott
Production Editor: Andrew Yackira

Photography ©2019 Biz Jones
Food styling by Erika Joyce
Author photo courtesy of ©Becca Batista

ISBN: Print 978-1-64152-719-4 | eBook 978-1-64152-720-0
R2

To my best friend and partner in crime,
my husband Jeremy, and to
our beautiful boys, Enzo and Luca!

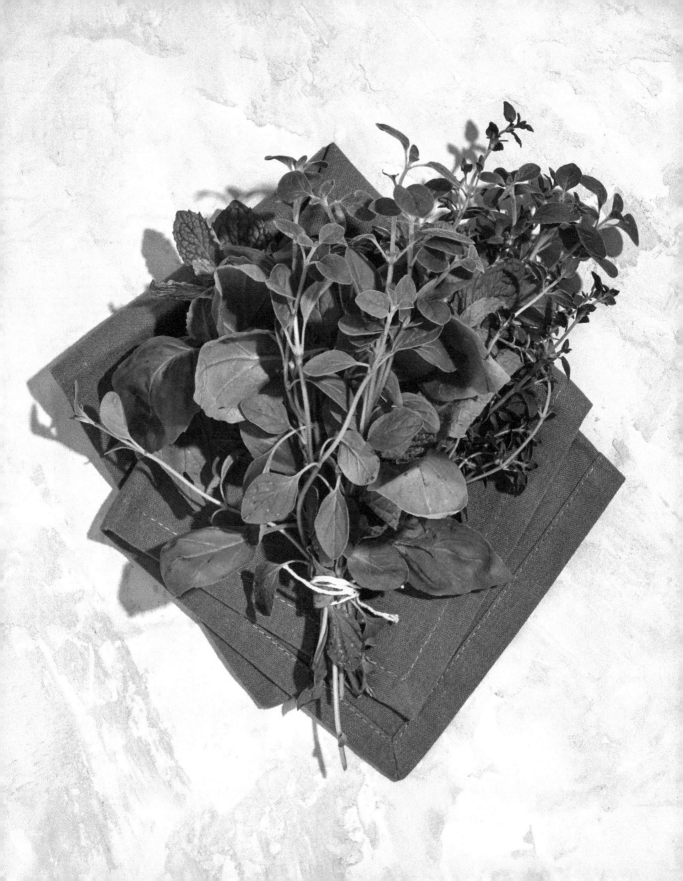

Contents

Introduction

I accidentally discovered the low-FODMAP diet back in 2013. It had been about three years since my symptoms of irritable bowel syndrome (IBS) started to greatly affect my quality of life. I visited several gastroenterologists, had breath tests, and a colonoscopy, and was diagnosed with IBS, but no one had an answer for what I should do next. When I asked one doctor how I could relieve my symptoms, I clearly remember him saying, "I don't know what to tell you."

I needed to know how to rid myself of the awful bloating, distention, constipation, and surprise emergency trips to the bathroom. I wanted to get back into running and competing, and I wanted to go out with friends without worrying if I was far from a bathroom.

After one very close call with humiliation in a public place, I went home and started researching online. That's when I found "FODMAP" and "IBS" in the same sentence. I was intrigued. As I learned about FODMAPs and which foods were the most troublesome, I started to consider the possible culprits for my own symptoms: the whole milk in my coffee; the times I had more than one small scoop of ice cream; the days I ate a whole apple, nectarine, or more than one piece of watermelon; the hummus or raw red onions in my beloved chicken salad.

I discovered that the low-FODMAP diet wasn't some fad but was actually backed by science, and more and more registered dietitians were praising it across the globe.

So, I decided to try the diet for myself. I created my grocery list of low-FODMAP foods and made everything from scratch (at the time, no certified low-FODMAP products were available in the United States). I recorded everything I ate in my food and symptom diary, and in a few days, I started to get results.

As I was making my way through the diet, I completed the Certified Nutritionist Consultant Program at the Natural Healing Institute of Naturopathy, Inc. Good nutrition was something I was already passionate about, but I wanted to understand the human digestive system and what could compromise digestion and overall health.

Following this diet has given me the freedom to do what I like to do and the confidence to eat and travel without worry, and I hope it will do the same for you.

The aim of this book is to provide simple, 30-minute low-FODMAP recipes to make the low-FODMAP diet easier to tackle. All the recipes in this book are entirely low-FODMAP and have been reviewed by Joanna Baker, APD, AN, RN, so you don't have to worry about triggering any FODMAP sensitivities.

Your low-FODMAP diet doesn't have to be devoid of fun or flavor! The ingredients used in this book are affordable, easy to find, and very simple to prepare. If you lead a busy life like me, you'll appreciate the ease of making these exciting and delicious recipes. Let's dig in!

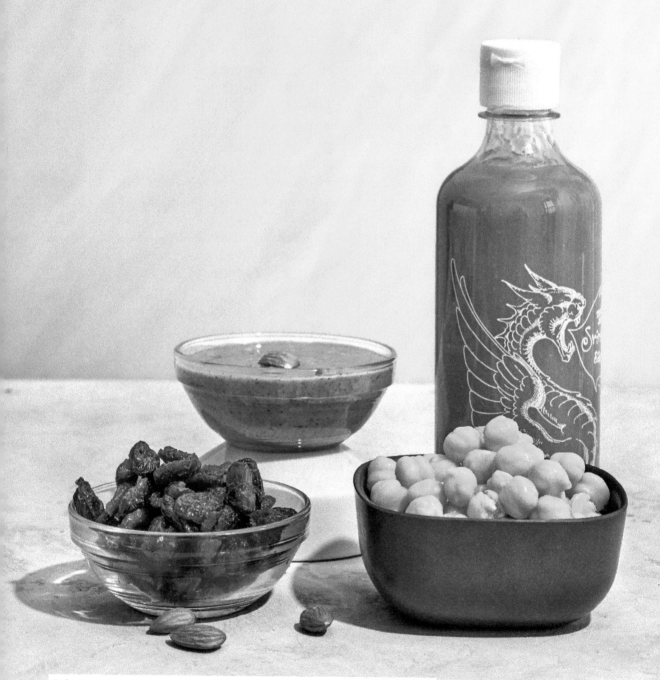

Dried cranberries, canned chickpeas, almond butter, and Sriracha sauce

CHAPTER 1

The Low-FODMAP Solution

Maybe you were recently diagnosed with IBS or you've thought all along that IBS was to blame for your discomfort. Maybe you've heard about the low-FODMAP diet from a friend or family member who cares and knows about your symptoms all too well. Whichever way you found this book, welcome! This diet may seem complicated, but once you learn the ropes and start feeling better, the time and effort you put in will be invaluable.

What are FODMAPs?

The foods we eat consist of proteins, carbs, and fats that are all essential for a balanced diet. However, certain carbohydrates in the FODMAP family can trigger IBS symptoms in some people. As a result, you may have heard someone say that all FODMAP-containing foods are "bad." The truth is that many FODMAP-containing foods are very healthy, which is why it's best to follow the diet to completion. Doing so will allow you to introduce unproblematic FODMAPs back into your diet and help keep your nutrition balanced.

FODMAPs are small molecules made up of short-chain carbohydrates (sugars and fibers) that are poorly absorbed in the small bowel and easily fermentable. After malabsorption, some FODMAPs draw water into the intestine by osmosis, and the increase in fluid and gas distends the bowel and can cause diarrhea.

Bacteria ferment FODMAPs as they pass into the large intestine, producing gases that can affect how the muscles in the wall of the bowel contract. This may trigger symptoms like bloating, flatulence, abdominal pain, and distention and increased forward movement (peristalsis) leading to diarrhea (IBS-D), constipation (IBS-C) or alternation of diarrhea and constipation (IBS-A/IBS-M).

You may be wondering what FODMAP stands for. Just talking about FODMAPs and trying to explain them to others is an adventure in itself. "Excuse me, FOD-what?" Let's spell out this tongue-twister for you:

F—Fermentable

O—Oligosaccharides

D—Disaccharides

M—Monosaccharides

A—And

P—Polyols

Here are the short-chain carbohydrates explained:

Fermentable. Fermentation is the process by which gut bacteria break down undigested FODMAPs to produce gases.

Oligosaccharides. These are made up of fructooligosaccharides (FOS) and galactooligosaccharides (GOS).

FOS are found in vegetables, fruits, and in plants like the flowering chicory root plant. Chicory is high-FODMAP, as is inulin, which can be extracted from the chicory root and isolated for use as a dietary fiber.

GOS are found in legumes, cashews, pistachios, soy milk made from whole soybeans, custard apple, oat milk, and other fruits and plants.

Disaccharides. The three most common disaccharides are sucrose, lactose, and maltose. In the low-FODMAP diet, it is the lactose that can be troublesome, specifically in high amounts. A half cup of custard has 6 grams of lactose and is high-FODMAP. A 1.5-ounce serving of Parmesan cheese has less than 1 gram of lactose and is low-FODMAP.

Monosaccharides. Monosaccharides consist of glucose, fructose, and galactose. In the low-FODMAP diet, fructose is what can be troublesome. An equal ratio of fructose to glucose is low-FODMAP. However, when the ratio of fructose to glucose is higher, it's considered excess fructose and high-FODMAP. Excess fructose is found in honey, apples, fresh figs, mango, asparagus, orange juice, rum, and more.

Polyols. These include certain sugar alcohols that are high-FODMAP and can create a laxative effect, causing gastrointestinal symptoms such as bloating, abdominal distention, and pain. The Polyols to avoid on the low-FODMAP diet include sorbitol, mannitol, maltitol, xylitol, and isomalt.

The average adult digestive tract is about 9 meters long, and it takes food about 6 to 24 hours from the time it is consumed to reach the colon, where FODMAPs are fermented, resulting in IBS symptoms. In other words, if you're experiencing IBS symptoms today, it could be due to something you ate earlier today or yesterday.

Why do FODMAPs cause digestive distress in some people?

Those with IBS or functional gastrointestinal disorders (FGIDs) may struggle with FODMAPs due to:

The way the muscles of the bowel respond (motility) to the distension. Food may move faster or slower through the gut.

Gut hypersensitivity to gas production. IBS individuals may produce more gas or have higher sensitivity to the gas they produce.

Bacterial overgrowth in the small intestine. Bacteria that are supposed to be located in the large intestine can sometimes move up to the narrower small intestine. This is called small intestinal bacterial overgrowth (SIBO).

FODMAPs are poorly absorbed in the small intestine and pass to the large intestine intact. Consequently, those FODMAPs may attract water into the digestive tract, leading to bloating, distention, and watery stools. In the large intestine the undigested FODMAPs are fermented by intestinal bacteria, resulting in the release of gases (hydrogen, carbon dioxide, and methane) that can lead to digestive distress.

THE ORIGINS OF THE LOW-FODMAP DIET

Peter Gibson, head of Luminal Gastroenterology Research at Monash University in Melbourne, Australia, set up the first Functional Gut Service in 2002, focusing on improvement for symptoms of IBS through dietary therapy. He recruited Dr. Jane Muir, a dietitian–scientist who had done seminal work in resistant starch and non-starch polysaccharides, and Dr. Sue Shepherd, a dietitian known for her clinical prowess in celiac disease. This partnership led to the development of the "new" FODMAP concept. They proposed that because all rapidly absorbed or indigestible short-chain carbohydrates could provoke IBS-like symptoms, restricting them simultaneously would more reliably reduce IBS symptoms than restricting one alone.

They first published their FODMAP concept in 2005. The hypothesis paper suggested that avoiding poorly digested short-chain carbohydrates would minimize stretching of the intestinal wall and reduce stimulation of the gut's nervous system. Not long after, the acronym, FODMAP, was created.

The Low-FODMAP Diet

What is the science behind the low-FODMAP diet? First of all, it's worth noting that there's no "one size fits all" approach to IBS. Each person with IBS can have different abdominal symptoms, and the degree to which they occur depends on how much malabsorption is experienced. The good news, however, is that by removing high-FODMAPs (Elimination Phase) and uncovering which foods trigger symptoms (Challenge Phase), the diet can truly be tailored to uncover each person's tolerance or FODMAP threshold.

IBS

IBS is a functional bowel disorder. The internal organs are normal, but the gut is not behaving in a normal way. Diagnosing IBS can be tricky; it can't be diagnosed by an X-ray or a blood test. Doctors use the Rome IV criteria for patients experiencing recurrent abdominal pain at least 1 day per week in the last 3 months on average, and that is associated with at least two of the following: increased or reduced pain from defecation, change in stool frequency, and change in stool form (appearance). In clinical trials, the low-FODMAP diet has been found to improve symptoms in up to 70 percent of patients with IBS.

IBD

Inflammatory Bowel Disease (IBD) includes ulcerative colitis and Crohn's disease. These are both autoimmune conditions that cause chronic inflammation along the digestive tract. If you are still experiencing symptoms even though your IBD is in remission, a low-FODMAP diet may help minimize gut discomfort and improve quality of life. The low-FODMAP diet has been shown to help with IBS-type symptoms when IBD is in remission by reducing gas production and osmotic activity in the intestines.

SIBO

Small intestinal bacterial overgrowth (SIBO) is not well understood and testing techniques are unreliable. If you think you have SIBO, it is best to discuss treatment with antibiotics with your doctor. There is no specific diet that is proven to treat SIBO, but many people have reported that a low-FODMAP diet has helped manage their symptoms.

What to Expect

Once you begin the low-FODMAP diet, you may notice a reduction in uncomfortable or painful symptoms that can adversely affect your social, professional, personal, and intimate life. Consequently, you may also experience renewed confidence. You may no longer need to be nervous about eating while traveling, attending an event, or before an important meeting. With the newfound knowledge of following the diet, you'll be less likely to have an accident or experience discomfort, pain, or residual stress.

Remember, it's best to speak with your physician before embarking on the low-FODMAP diet.

GLUTEN FREE?

The low-FODMAP diet is not a gluten-free diet. Gluten is a protein found in wheat, barley, and rye; FODMAPs are the carbohydrates found in these grains. These different molecules are often found in the same foods. Gluten-free foods do not contain wheat, so many gluten-free foods can be consumed on the low-FODMAP diet as long as they don't contain other high-FODMAP ingredients.

Unless you have celiac disease, food sensitivities, or allergies, switching to a gluten-free diet without the direction of a physician is not suggested. Some still believe that gluten-free diets are "healthier," but that isn't the case as many gluten-free foods lack essential B vitamins and minerals.

If you have celiac disease, a low-FODMAP diet may help reduce your gastrointestinal symptoms. Some people with celiac disease can also have problems with other FODMAPs.

What to Lose (High-FODMAP) and What to Choose (Low-FODMAP)

IBS patients are often faced with options and brands that don't typically cater to their sensitivities. This list can help with making easy food substitutions.

What to Lose

Garlic

Onion

Agave syrup

Clover honey

Inulin fiber

Blueberry jam

Baked beans

Almonds

Cashews

Chickpeas, sprouted

Tofu, silken

Corn, kernels, canned

Blackberries

Apple, dried

Guava, unripe

Bread, pumpernickel

Bread, gluten-free sweetened with molasses

Couscous, wheat

Flour, barley

Pasta, wheat

Sausage seasoned with garlic

Rotisserie chicken, store-bought

Canned tomatoes with garlic or onion

Store-bought salad dressing with garlic, onion, milk products, honey, agave, high-FODMAP fruits or vegetables

Ketchup

Salsa with garlic and onion

Pasta sauce with onion and garlic

Cream sauce

Whey protein concentrate

Espresso with regular cow's milk

Chamomile tea

Wine—sticky, dessert

What to Choose

Asafetida powder by Casa de Sante™

Leek leaves

Maple syrup

Honey, 1 teaspoon*

Psyllium husk fiber

Strawberry jam

Butter beans, canned, ¼ cup

Peanuts, 32

Brazil nuts

Chickpeas, canned

Tofu, firm

Corn, baby, canned

Blueberries

Banana chips, dried

Guava, ripe

Bread, spelt, sourdough

Bread, gluten-free sweetened with cane sugar

Couscous, gluten-free made from maize flour

Better Batter all-purpose flour mix gluten-free

Pasta, wheat, ½ cup or gluten-free, 1 cup

Plain sausage seasoned with salt and pepper

Plain chicken cutlets

Canned tomatoes with tomato juice, calcium chloride, citric acid

Homemade salad dressing

Homemade ketchup or certified low-FODMAP ketchup by Fody™

Homemade salsa or Casa de Sante™ Salsa

Homemade sauce or Prego® Sensitive Recipe

Make a roux with butter, low-FODMAP flour, lactose-free milk, and Parmesan cheese

NAKED Nutrition® unflavored pea protein powder

Espresso with lactose-free cow's milk

Green tea

Wine—red, white, sweet, sparkling

*Indicates this food can become moderate to high in FODMAPs. Always follow suggested servings. Alternatively, if you are using a food that could potentially become moderate to high in FODMAPs and you are not sure about the weight or volume, you can always use an electronic food scale.

This list does not include all low-FODMAP foods. Please consult your low-FODMAP diet app for a full list of foods that have been tested for FODMAPs and review their servings and ratings (low, moderate, or high in FODMAPs). Be aware that new foods are added every so often, but some foods have sometimes been retested or removed so it's important to use your app and check for app updates.

For an expanded list of Low-FODMAP foods that you can stock your kitchen with and safely enjoy, see page 145.

A Balanced Diet

Can you think back to a day where you felt a little "off"? Your body and mind felt sluggish. With each daily task, your energy waned. What was making you feel like you were running like an old VCR? Be honest—was it because you'd been cheating on your health with foods devoid of nutrition? It's okay; we all get off track sometimes, and that experience is a great lesson on why nutritious foods are important for your health.

Nutritious foods can improve your mood, boost energy, keep you regular, prevent disease, help maintain a healthy weight, keep mental health in check, and boost your immune system. Did you know that your bowel is a secondary lymphatic organ yet it contains an incredible 70 to 80 percent of the body's immune cells? So, you can imagine how healthy food choices may improve the health of your gut!

In addition to choosing nutritious foods, it's also important to make every plate balanced. A balanced diet means you can enjoy a wide variety of nutrients to support your body's various needs. And when it comes to following the low-FODMAP diet, a balanced diet is especially key.

The Importance of Portions

One of the keys to success when following the low-FODMAP diet is to follow listed servings so you can balance your daily meals with the right portions and avoid accidentally consuming too many FODMAPs in the course of a day.

Here are three things to keep in mind:

1. Some foods come with low-FODMAP servings as well as moderate- and high-FODMAP servings. For example, half a cob of sweet corn is low-FODMAP, but just a quarter more becomes moderate in the Polyol sorbitol, and a whole cob is high-FODMAP.
2. Avoid FODMAP stacking. Some foods come with low-FODMAP servings but may also have "upper limit" servings.
3. If a food comes with a moderate- to high-FODMAP serving, it might be okay for you to consume one low-FODMAP serving per sitting more than one time per day. Wait three to four hours in between each serving. *(Keeping a food and symptom diary can help you understand which foods and quantities are best for you.)*

Why Not FODMAP-free?

Consuming a wide variety of nutrients in your diet is essential to overall health, and cutting out all high-FODMAPs for an extended period of time can actually be harmful.

Although certain FODMAPs can cause digestive distress, some are very beneficial to our health. FODMAPs can help protect the immune system and fight off disease. That's why it is critical to follow the diet all the way through each phase and uncover your triggers. That way, you may be able to bring back in some FODMAP-containing foods like Jerusalem artichoke, apples, asparagus, barley, chicory root, and leek bulbs. Who knows, maybe you'll find you can incorporate large or small amounts of onions or garlic.

I'M VEGAN/VEGETARIAN—IS THE LOW-FODMAP DIET RIGHT FOR ME?

The low-FODMAP diet excludes many different kinds of fruits, vegetables, plant-based proteins, and dairy foods. So, if you're vegan or vegetarian, it can be easy to become deficient in nutrients like fiber, calcium, and vitamin D. Kate Scarlata, RD and FODMAP expert, recommends that vegans (and anyone with multiple dietary restrictions) spend no more than two weeks in the Elimination Phase to avoid nutritional shortcomings.

For protein, vegans often rely on legumes that are high-FODMAP, so they may struggle to get enough protein and vitamin B_{12} during the Elimination Phase. Strict vegans may be at risk for multiple vitamin and mineral deficiencies, including some amino acids the body uses to make protein. A multivitamin can help cover your bases (remember to check with your doctor or dietitian before taking any supplements). Some great vegan sources of low-FODMAP protein include extra-firm tofu, tempeh, and edamame.

It's a little easier for vegetarians to follow the diet because they have more choices for protein. Be sure to get enough iron from leafy low-FODMAP greens, and don't forget sources of healthy fats like flax seeds, nuts, and avocado (watch servings). And lastly, be sure to try various low-FODMAP vegetables.

How to Say Goodbye to Trigger Foods

Start your food and symptom diary and keep track of all you eat and drink so that you and your dietitian can see what works best. Look through your pantry, refrigerator, and freezer, and start reading all food labels. Learn about the different high-FODMAP alternatives you can eat (see the chart on page 9) and make a grocery list with your chosen high-FODMAP alternatives.

As with all elimination diets, or any diet for that matter, eliminating foods you regularly eat can throw a wrench into your regular routine. You may have grown accustomed to buying the same foods at the grocery store, or eating lunch at the café near work, or simply eating whatever you want. Just remember, the low-FODMAP diet is temporary and can have outstanding results for your gut health.

Plan your meals for the week, and find time to prep ingredients and snacks so you never go hangry. Doing so will keep you prepared, give you peace of mind, and help you avoid mistakes. But if you do make a mistake, don't beat yourself up!

Say goodbye to trigger foods and hello to your low-FODMAP journey!

Allium Flavors	
Garlic	Garlic-Infused Oil (page 134), asafetida powder
Onion	Leek leaves, green tips of onions, asafetida powder, onion and Shallot-Infused Oil (page 136)
Lactose and Dairy Alternatives	
Regular cow's milk	Lactose-free full-fat milk
Regular cow's milk yogurt	Plain lactose-free yogurt, 6 ounces Greek yogurt (strained)
Buttermilk	½ cup dairy-free milk plus 1 tablespoon lemon juice. Whisk well. Leave the mixture to coagulate at room temperature for about 10 minutes.

Lactose and Dairy Alternatives	
Kefir	Lactose-free kefir
Coconut milk with inulin	Coconut milk without inulin
Soy milk made from soybeans	Soy milk made from soy protein

Beans	
Borlotti beans	Butter beans, canned, ¼ cup
Cashews	Cashews, activated, 10 nuts
Chickpeas, sprouted	Chickpeas, canned (drained and rinsed) ¼ cup
Lentil burger	Homemade Lentil Burgers (page 67)
Mung beans, boiled (¼ cup is low)	Mung beans, sprouted, ⅔ cup
Tofu, silken	Tofu, plain or firm, drained

Sweeteners	
Clover honey, 1 teaspoon	Regular honey, 1 teaspoon
Agave syrup	Pure maple syrup, 1 tablespoon
Milk chocolate	Dark chocolate
Coconut sugar	Light brown sugar

Spiciness	
Hot sauce	Sriracha hot chili sauce
Chili, red, 28 grams or less	Chili, green, 28 grams or more
Chili, chipotle (dried)	Homemade low-FODMAP chipotle in adobo sauce
Salsa	Certified low-FODMAP salsa

ELIMINATION AND REINTRODUCTION

It's important to avoid hovering in the Elimination and Reintroduction (i.e., Challenge) Phases of the diet. Your body needs a wide variety of nutrients from all five food groups, so moving on to the Modified Phase is crucial.

In the Elimination Phase, high-FODMAP foods are omitted from your diet for 2 to 6 weeks (unless your doctor or dietician is supervising your progress and has advised a longer period). You still have many options from all five food groups during this phase so that you can maintain healthy nutrition. In the Reintroduction Phase, you'll challenge 8 to 10 high-FODMAP foods for 8 to 12 weeks. Reintroducing one food at a time from each FODMAP group with small, medium, and large(-ish) serving sizes will give you a better understanding of your FODMAP tolerance.

The Modified Phase is when you've figured out your "FODMAP threshold"— the types of FODMAPs that affect you most, and those you can or can't tolerate—and come up with the best ongoing diet for yourself based on your personal triggers.

Discussing a complete plan for Elimination and Reintroduction is outside the scope of this book, but we highly recommend working with a FODMAP-trained dietitian or signing up for The Low-FODMAP Diet Beginner's Course (an online course hosted on Teachable: https://fodmap-life.teachable.com/p/low-fodmap -diet-beginners-course).

Preparing Your Kitchen and Pantry

If you desire flavor and want variety in the dishes you make, I highly suggest getting your pantry ready before you start the low-FODMAP diet. Listed below is a sampling of essential low-FODMAP items that can be purchased at your local grocery store, or you can buy them online.

Canned and Bottled Items

- Chickpeas
- Tomatoes (without added high-FODMAPs)
- Jam, strawberry
- Low-FODMAP ketchup
- Low-FODMAP barbecue sauce
- Low-FODMAP salsa

- Mayonnaise
- Mustard
- Soy sauce
- Sriracha sauce
- Tomato paste
- Worcestershire sauce

Pantry Items

- Asafetida powder
- Cayenne pepper
- Chili powder
- Cinnamon
- Cumin
- Dried cranberries
- Freshly ground black pepper
- Garlic-Infused Oil (page 134)
- Maple syrup
- Mayonnaise
- Peanut butter or almond butter
- Oats

- Oils—avocado, canola, coconut, olive, sesame
- Oregano
- Paprika
- Polenta or low-FODMAP pasta
- Quinoa
- Rice
- Rosemary
- Salt—kosher salt, sea salt
- Thyme
- Vinegars—apple cider vinegar, red wine vinegar, rice wine vinegar

FINDING FODMAPS IN INGREDIENT LISTS

It can be tricky to search for high-FODMAPs on food labels, but once you know what to look for, this task will be a breeze. Believe it or not, over-the-counter medicine and medications can also contain high-FODMAPs. If you've found your medicine or medications contain high-FODMAPs, please do not stop taking them until you've consulted with your physician. They may know of alternatives for you.

The following list represents the type of high-FODMAPs most likely to be found on food labels:

OLIGOSACCHARIDES

- Garlic, garlic powder, garlic extract
- Onion, onion powder, or onion extract
- "Natural flavors" or "spices" that could be onion or garlic
- Inulin, chicory root, chicory root fiber
- Fructooligosaccharides
- Wheat, barley, or rye when a main ingredient

DISACCHARIDES

- Lactose
- Milk
- Nonfat dry milk
- Milk protein concentrate (in higher amounts)
- Whey protein concentrate
- Whey protein hydrolysate (High-FODMAP unless labeled lactose-free)

MONOSACCHARIDES

- High-fructose corn syrup
- Fructose
- Fructose-glucose syrup
- Crystalline fructose
- Honey
- Agave
- Isoglucose

POLYOLS

- Sorbitol
- Mannitol
- Maltitol
- Xylitol
- Isomalt

In my own life, I am very busy running my business and caring for my family, so I need recipes that are quick to make but also family approved. That is why I have come up with 101 low-FODMAP recipes that can be made in about 30 minutes!

Throughout the recipes, I list various tips to help you safely cook low-FODMAP. When I have used an ingredient within a recipe that could be potentially moderate- to high-FODMAP, I will provide a **FODMAP tip** as a warning. I also list **Ingredient tips**, **Make-ahead tips**, **Substitution tips**, and **Preparation tips**. Please read the tips before you begin each recipe; they will help you buy the right foods, use the correct servings, and save time.

Looking for a smoothie, perhaps some hot chocolate, or something tasty to start your day? Head over to **Chapter 2**, where I cover smoothies, beverages, and breakfasts. **Chapter 3** will introduce you to delicious sides and salads. From appetizers to soups, vegetable side dishes, and salads, there's something here for everyone.

Vegans, vegetarians, and omnivores alike will love **Chapter 4** as there are so many choices, from basic to exotic. **Chapter 5** contains some of my favorite fish and seafood meals. If you're in the mood for poultry or meat, cozy up in the kitchen with some of the exciting recipes in **Chapter 6**.

And how about something sweet? From cheese to fruit and chocolate, **Chapter 7** has many sweet and delicious options. **Chapter 8** is where you'll find recipes for making your own broths, stocks, sauces, oils, and dressings that are very easy and will make your dishes much tastier! Note that all of the recipes found in this book are entirely low-FODMAP and follow low-FODMAP diet guidelines. Unless otherwise stated, one serving from each recipe is equal to one low-FODMAP serving.

Icon indicates
potentially
moderate- to
high-FODMAP

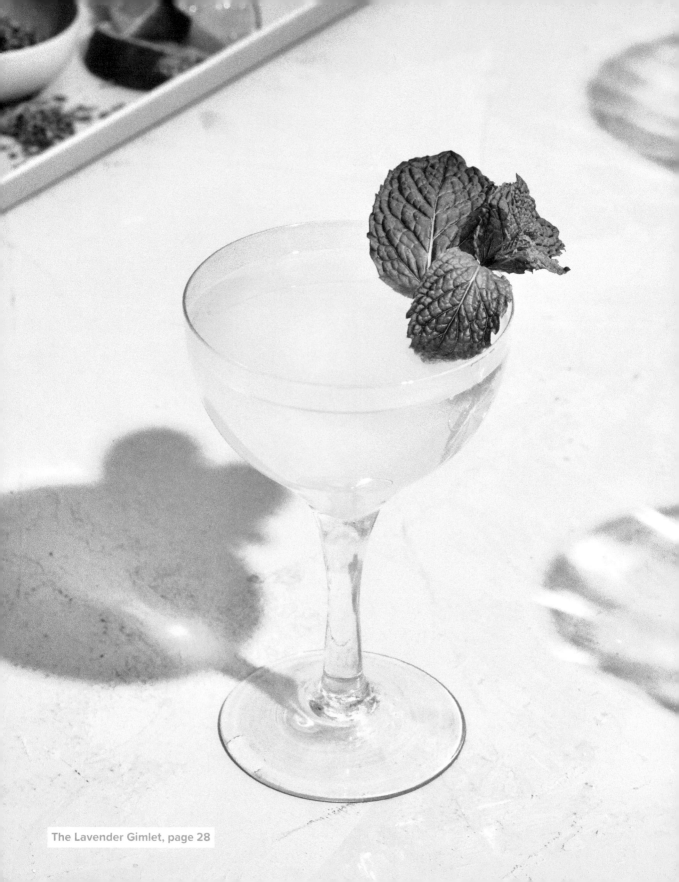

The Lavender Gimlet, page 28

CHAPTER 2

Smoothies, Beverages, and Breakfasts

Almond Pineapple Anti-Inflammatory Smoothie

Prep time: 10 minutes, plus overnight to soak / Serves: 1

DAIRY-FREE, VEGETARIAN, UNDER 20 MINUTES

This smoothie recipe is wonderful for times when IBS inflammation strikes. It contains anti-inflammatory ingredients to help soothe your gut. When you feel like your gut could use a helping hand, try this smoothie on an empty stomach and sip slowly.

10 raw almonds, soaked overnight and drained

1½ cups water

½ cup fresh pineapple

½ medium frozen firm banana, peeled

1 medium carrot, peeled

½ tablespoon freshly squeezed lemon juice

½ teaspoon ground turmeric

1 teaspoon grated fresh ginger

½ teaspoon ground cinnamon

1 teaspoon honey

1. Blend the almonds and water together until very smooth, about 1 minute.

2. Add the pineapple, banana, carrot, lemon juice, turmeric, ginger, cinnamon, and honey and blend until smooth.

3. Add more lemon juice, ginger, or cinnamon to taste.

Substitution tip: Make this smoothie vegan by using up to 1 tablespoon of maple syrup in place of honey.

Per serving: Calories: 209; Total fat: 7g; Total carbs: 38g; Fiber: 6g; Sugar: 23g; Protein: 4g; Sodium: 43mg

Chai Smoothie

Prep time: 2 minutes / Serves: 1

DAIRY-FREE, VEGETARIAN, QUICK-PREP, UNDER 10 MINUTES

Chai is high-FODMAP, but with this delicious smoothie, I've created the essence of chai with the right combination of warm spice and sweetness. Have it for breakfast or as a late-morning snack.

1 medium frozen firm banana, peeled

½ teaspoon ground ginger

½ teaspoon ground cinnamon

¼ teaspoon ground cardamom

¼ teaspoon ground nutmeg

1 teaspoon honey

½ teaspoon pure vanilla extract

1 tablespoon almond butter

1 cup unsweetened almond milk

Put the banana, ginger, cinnamon, cardamom, nutmeg, honey, vanilla, almond butter, and almond milk into a blender and blend until smooth.

FODMAP tip: *Honey is allowed on the low-FODMAP diet, but only at 1 teaspoon per serving. Be sure to only use regular honey for this recipe and not clover honey.*

Per serving: Calories: 265; Total fat: 13g; Total carbs: 36g; Fiber: 6g; Sugar: 19g; Protein: 6g; Sodium: 183mg

Banana Protein Power Shake

Prep time: 2 minutes / **Serves:** 1

VEGETARIAN, QUICK-PREP, UNDER 10 MINUTES

This shake is packed with protein and is my favorite post-workout shake. The yogurt, protein powder, and low-FODMAP ingredients will make you feel full and satisfied but not bloated. This is also a good smoothie to have for breakfast. Just remember to sit down and drink this smoothie slowly!

1 cup plain unsweetened almond milk

6 ounces strained Greek yogurt

1 cup spinach

1 serving unflavored pea protein powder

1 medium frozen firm banana, peeled

⅛ teaspoon ground cinnamon

Put the almond milk, yogurt, spinach, protein powder, banana, and cinnamon into a blender and blend until smooth.

FODMAP tip: *Make sure the Greek yogurt you choose has been strained. This process lowers the lactose and makes the yogurt low-FODMAP. Stick to 6 ounces or less.*

Ingredient tip: Any low-FODMAP protein powder will work with this shake.

Per serving: Calories: 422; Total fat: 12g; Total carbs: 34g; Fiber: 6g; Sugar: 19g; Protein: 44g; Sodium: 432mg

Peanut Butter and Coffee Smoothie

Prep time: 2 minutes / **Serves:** 1

VEGETARIAN, QUICK-PREP, UNDER 10 MINUTES

Who doesn't love peanut butter any time of the day? This is a yummy way to incorporate your morning cup of Joe with breakfast. Instant coffee with caffeine and decaf coffee are low-FODMAP, but be mindful of the milk you add.

½ **cup ice, plus more as needed**

¾ **cup unsweetened low-FODMAP milk of choice**

¼ **cup brewed regular instant coffee, chilled (made with 2 heaped teaspoons of grounds)**

1 **tablespoon ground coffee**

1 **tablespoon natural peanut butter**

½ **teaspoon pure vanilla extract**

1 **medium frozen firm banana, peeled**

1 **teaspoon honey**

1. Combine the ice, milk, and instant coffee in a blender first, then add the ground coffee, peanut butter, vanilla, banana, and honey and blend until smooth.

2. If you'd like a thicker consistency, add ¼ cup of ice at a time and blend.

FODMAP tip: *Always check the labels on peanut butter or other nut butters for high-FODMAPs like agave, honey, and inulin. Honey is allowed on the low-FODMAP diet, but only at 1 teaspoon per serving. Clover honey is allowed only at ½ teaspoon per serving.*

Per serving: Calories: 246; Total fat: 11g; Total carbs: 33g; Fiber: 4g; Sugar: 19g; Protein: 7g; Sodium: 140mg

Green and Fruity Protein Smoothie

Prep time: 2 minutes / Serves: 1

VEGETARIAN, QUICK-PREP, UNDER 10 MINUTES

This smoothie mixes two delicious fruits together that equal one low-FODMAP serving. When making any smoothie, it's important to only use low-FODMAP fruits that equal one serving. Be mindful of nut butters and the correct serving sizes, and add some maple syrup and stevia powder for an extra touch of sweetness.

1 cup unsweetened
    almond milk

1 cup baby
    spinach, packed

½ medium frozen firm
    banana, peeled

1 small kiwi, peeled and
    cut into chunks

1 tablespoon
    almond butter

1 serving low-FODMAP
    protein powder

1 teaspoon maple
    syrup (optional)

Pinch stevia powder
    (optional)

Put the almond milk, spinach, banana, kiwi, almond butter, protein powder, maple syrup (if using), and stevia (if using) into a blender and blend until smooth.

FODMAP tip: *Be sure to stick to 1 tablespoon of almond butter per meal to avoid consuming moderate- to high-FODMAPs.*

Per serving: Calories: 395; Total fat: 18g; Total carbs: 33g; Fiber: 8g; Sugar: 15g; Protein: 30g; Sodium: 341mg

Red-Hot Chili Hot Chocolate

Prep time: 2 minutes / **Cook time:** 6 minutes / **Serves:** 2

QUICK-PREP, UNDER 10 MINUTES

Curling up with a book or a movie? Just come back from a run, hike, or skiing on a winter day? Take time out for yourself and sail away with this sultry, smooth, and slightly spicy hot chocolate. Most store-bought hot chocolate contains lactose or other milk products so I always make my own at home and find doing so is a very fun process.

2 ounces dark chocolate morsels

1 tablespoon unsweetened cocoa powder

1 tablespoon sugar or 1½ packets Pyure® Organic Stevia

⅛ teaspoon ancho chili powder

1 cup whole lactose-free cow's milk

2 tablespoons canned coconut cream

¼ teaspoon ground cinnamon

½ teaspoon pure vanilla extract

⅔ cup mini marshmallows, divided (optional)

½ cup whipped cream, divided (optional)

1. Set a small saucepot over medium-low heat and whisk together the dark chocolate, cocoa powder, sugar, and chili powder. Once the ingredients begin to melt, slowly whisk in the milk, coconut cream, cinnamon, and vanilla. Bring to a simmer for 5 minutes.

2. Remove from the heat and ladle into 2 mugs. Serve immediately with marshmallows and/or whipped cream (if using).

Cooking tip: The chocolate melts very fast. To prevent burning, be sure to have all the ingredients, measuring spoons, and cups ready to go.

Substitution tip: Forgo the chili powder if you prefer hot chocolate without the spice.

Ingredient tip: Make sure you buy chili powder made from dried ancho chiles, and avoid any chili powder that contains other "spices" like garlic.

Per serving: Calories: 341; Total fat: 19g; Total carbs: 37g; Fiber: 5g; Sugar: 30g; Protein: 7g; Sodium: 70mg

The Lavender Gimlet

Prep time: 2 minutes / Serves: 1

5 INGREDIENTS OR LESS, ALCOHOLIC, DAIRY-FREE, NUT-FREE, VEGETARIAN, QUICK-PREP, UNDER 10 MINUTES

If you want to try something new and give your low-FODMAP cocktails some flavor, Sonoma Syrup Co.'s simple syrups are wonderful for both nonalcoholic and alcoholic drinks. Since alcohol can be a gut irritant and throw off your results for the diet, it is recommended to drink occasionally or for special events.

2 tablespoons gin

1 tablespoon Sonoma Syrup Co. Lavender Infused Simple Syrup

1 teaspoon lime juice

½ cup ice

Lime wheel or 1 sprig mint, for garnish (optional)

1. Pour the gin, simple syrup, lime juice, and ice into a shaker and shake until chilled. Strain into a chilled glass and garnish with a lime wheel or mint (if using).

2. If you don't have a shaker, combine everything in a glass and stir vigorously with a long cocktail spoon. Another option is to put all the ingredients (except for the garnish) in a blender for a frozen lavender gimlet.

Preparation tip: Make your own simple syrup by combining 1 cup of sugar and 1 cup of water and stirring consistently in a saucepot over medium heat. Once the sugar has dissolved, remove from the heat. Immediately stir in a few tablespoons of culinary lavender buds (or other ingredients such as culinary rosemary and clove, fresh mint, ginger, pepper, etc.) and cover to steep. Once cool, drain the lavender buds through a mesh strainer. Store in an airtight container in the refrigerator for 1 to 2 weeks. Plain simple syrup can stay fresh for up to 4 weeks.

Per serving: Calories: 101; Total fat: 0g; Total carbs: 8g; Fiber: 1g; Sugar: 7g; Protein: 0g; Sodium: 1mg

Thai Iced Tea

Prep time: 2 minutes / Cook time: 5 minutes / Serves: 2

DAIRY-FREE, NUT-FREE, VEGETARIAN, QUICK-PREP, UNDER 10 MINUTES

When my husband and I were living in California, there were many places that served Thai tea. It's definitely a "treat" I like to enjoy on occasion. Despite not containing high-FODMAP ingredients, this drink is tasty, great for entertaining, and can be a nice dessert. My version of Thai tea does not contain food coloring or high-FODMAPs such as condensed or evaporated milk, and it's much lower in sugar. สนุก! (Enjoy!)

2 cups water

2 organic black tea bags

1 tablespoon sugar, or 1½ packets Pyure® Organic Stevia

1 star anise pod

1 cardamom pod or ⅛ teaspoon ground cardamom

2 whole cloves

½ cinnamon stick

¼ teaspoon pure vanilla extract

Ice

½ cup unsweetened canned coconut milk, divided

1. Boil the water in a saucepan or a glass measuring cup. Once the water comes to a boil, steep the tea bags, sugar, star anise, cardamom, cloves, cinnamon stick, and vanilla for 5 minutes.

2. Strain the ingredients in a mesh strainer over another glass measuring cup or a medium mixing bowl.

3. Fill 2 glasses with ice and pour in the tea mixture ¾ of the way. Fill the rest of both glasses with the coconut milk. Taste and adjust with more sugar or spice if desired. Enjoy!

FODMAP tip: *Be sure the canned coconut milk you buy does not include inulin.*

Make-ahead tip: If you have the time, allow the tea bags to steep for about 2 hours for a bolder flavor.

Preparation tip: Add more sugar if you desire or use stevia. Up to 1 teaspoon of powdered stevia is low-FODMAP.

Ingredient tip: Cardamom pods are ideal for this recipe, but ground cardamom works as well.

Per serving: Calories: 162; Total fat: 14g; Total carbs: 9g; Fiber: 1g; Sugar: 8g; Protein: 1g; Sodium: 9mg

Peanut Butter & Jam Oatmeal

Prep time: 2 minutes / **Cook time:** 10 minutes / **Serves:** 1

VEGETARIAN, QUICK-PREP, UNDER 20 MINUTES

If you've only made oatmeal in the microwave, you've been missing out! Oats cook better over the stovetop and become tenderer and soak up the flavors from the rest of the ingredients. Oats are a great choice when you want to feel fuller longer. Be sure to pay attention to the serving size for instant or rolled oats as different processing methods can yield varying levels of FODMAPs.

¼ cup low-FODMAP milk of choice

½ cup old-fashioned rolled oats

⅛ teaspoon kosher salt

1 tablespoon strawberry jam

1 tablespoon peanut butter

1 tablespoon crushed and roasted peanuts (optional)

1. In a medium saucepan over high heat, bring the milk to a boil. Quickly stir in the oats and salt, reduce the heat to low, and simmer until the oats are tender and creamy, 5 minutes. (You can make the oats creamier by adding in 1 tablespoon of milk at a time until the desired level of creaminess is reached.)

2. Stir in the jam and peanut butter and let warm, 1 minute. Transfer the oatmeal to a bowl and top with the roasted peanuts (if using) and serve immediately.

FODMAP tip: When buying strawberry jam, make sure it does not contain high-FODMAP ingredients. If you would like to use 1 tablespoon of a different nut butter, be sure to avoid cashew and pistachio nut butters as they are all high-FODMAP.

Substitution tip: You can sub out peanut butter for sunflower seed butter or 1 tablespoon of almond butter, which is only low-FODMAP at 1 tablespoon.

Per serving: Calories: 341; Total fat: 12g; Total carbs: 49g; Fiber: 6g; Sugar: 2g; Protein: 10g; Sodium: 346mg

Sweet Potato Chocolate Pancakes

Prep time: 10 minutes / Cook time: 30 minutes / Serves: 6 (12 pancakes)

VEGETARIAN

Eating low-FODMAP doesn't mean you can't enjoy breakfast treats like pancakes. But forget about plain old pancakes: these sweet potato pancakes with chocolate and nuts are just the thing for any morning when you want to treat yourself. Baking these pancakes in a pan means less time standing over the stove and more time to put your feet up and relax.

Nonstick cooking spray

1 large sweet potato

2 eggs, beaten

1½ cups low-FODMAP milk

¼ cup butter, melted

1½ cups gluten-free low-FODMAP all-purpose flour with xanthan gum (I prefer Better Batter All-Purpose Flour Mix)

3½ teaspoons baking powder

1 teaspoon kosher salt

½ teaspoon ground nutmeg

½ cup chopped pecans or walnuts

½ cup dark chocolate chips

1. Preheat the oven to 375°F. Prepare a (13-by-18-inch) half baking sheet with parchment paper and spray lightly with the nonstick cooking spray. Set aside.

2. Cook the sweet potato in the microwave for 4 minutes. Flip it over and cook for another 3 to 4 minutes, until a fork can pierce completely through the potato. Carefully cut the potato in half. Using a tablespoon, scoop out and measure 1 cup of sweet potato and put in a medium bowl. Mash until very soft. Add the eggs, milk, and butter.

3. In another medium bowl, sift together the flour, baking powder, salt, and nutmeg. Add the sweet potato mixture into the flour mixture and mix well to form a batter.

4. In a small bowl, combine the nuts and chocolate chips and mix together.

5. Transfer the pancake batter to the prepared baking sheet. Then evenly sprinkle the nuts and chocolate chips across the top of the batter.

6. Bake for 18 to 20 minutes, until set.

7. Allow to cool for 5 minutes before slicing into 12 pancakes.

Continued ▶

Sweet Potato Chocolate Pancakes
continued

FODMAP tip: When it comes to a great all-purpose flour made with low-FODMAP ingredients, I prefer Better Batter All-Purpose Flour Mix. It already contains xanthan gum and is free of the top 11 allergens.

Ingredient tip: When buying sweet potato for this recipe, buy one large sweet potato or two medium sweet potatoes. This will help ensure you have enough to measure out for the recipe.

Preparation tip: If you have only a larger baking sheet (21-by-15-inch), the batter will be thick enough to stay in place if you just smooth it over three-quarters of the way.

Per serving (2 pancakes): Calories: 374; Total fat: 21g; Total carbs: 42g; Fiber: 2g; Sugar: 7g; Protein: 6g; Sodium: 297mg

Lemon Coconut Pancakes

Prep time: 5 minutes / **Cook time:** 20 minutes / **Serves:** 4 (8 pancakes)

DAIRY-FREE, VEGETARIAN, QUICK-PREP, UNDER 30 MINUTES

Lemon and shredded coconut make for a very subtle, delicious taste in these pancakes. The tart and sweet flavors will delight you! Indulge in these pancakes for yourself or make them for friends and family at your next social brunch.

1 room temperature egg or Flax Egg (page 143)

2 tablespoons granulated sugar

2 tablespoons vegetable oil

1 teaspoon pure vanilla extract

2 tablespoons freshly squeezed lemon juice

2 teaspoons lemon zest

1 cup gluten-free low-FODMAP all-purpose flour with xanthan gum (I prefer Better Batter All-Purpose Flour Mix)

1 tablespoon baking powder

½ cup dried shredded unsweetened coconut

¼ teaspoon kosher salt

¾ cup rice, almond, or macadamia milk

Maple syrup, for topping (optional)

1. Grease and preheat an 11-inch nonstick griddle or pan to 375°F.

2. In a large bowl, whisk together the egg, sugar, vegetable oil, vanilla, lemon juice, and lemon zest.

3. Over another bowl, pass the flour through a fine sieve. Add the baking powder, coconut, and salt. Whisk to combine.

4. Slowly whisk the egg mixture into the flour mixture. Stir in the milk and mix until all the ingredients are smooth but not overly smooth (lumps are okay).

5. Turn the preheated griddle down to 365°F and pour or scoop the batter onto the pan, using about ¼ cup of batter each time. Cook until bubbly on top and golden on bottom, about 4 minutes. Flip and cook until golden on the bottom, about 2 more minutes. Top with maple syrup (if using).

FODMAP tip: *Dried and shredded coconut is low-FODMAP at a ½-cup serving.*

Per serving (2 pancakes): Calories: 263; Total fat: 13g; Total carbs: 32g; Fiber: 5g; Sugar: 7g; Protein: 5g; Sodium: 237mg

Egg-and-Cheese Stuffed Baked Potato

Prep time: 2 minutes / Cook time: 15 minutes / Serves: 1

NUT-FREE, VEGETARIAN, QUICK-PREP, UNDER 20 MINUTES

When your morning is filled with many tasks, this meal will keep you going strong until lunchtime. Filling and warm, the potato and egg are super easy to make, and you may already have most of the ingredients in your kitchen.

1 medium unpeeled sweet potato

1 teaspoon butter

1 large egg, beaten

1 teaspoon extra-virgin olive oil

Kosher salt

Freshly ground black pepper

1 tablespoon shredded cheddar or Monterey Jack cheese

1 teaspoon chopped scallions, green parts only

1 tablespoon regular sour cream (optional)

1. Prick the sweet potato several times with a fork. Cook it on full power in the microwave for 5 minutes. Turn it over and continue to cook for 5 more minutes. Carefully cut in half lengthwise.

2. In a nonstick skillet on medium-high heat, melt the butter and scramble the egg until cooked through.

3. Take half of the baked potato and scoop out about 2 tablespoons of potato. Drizzle with the olive oil and season with salt and pepper. Stuff the potato with the scrambled egg. Top with the shredded cheese and scallions, and finish with the sour cream (if using).

FODMAP tip: *Only up to 2 tablespoons of regular sour cream is low-FODMAP, which is plenty for this recipe.*

Per serving: Calories: 322; Total fat: 14g; Total carbs: 38g; Fiber: 4g; Sugar: 2g; Protein: 12g; Sodium: 308mg

Bacon and Cheese Breakfast Wrap

Prep time: 2 minutes / Cook time: 15 minutes / Serves: 1

NUT-FREE, QUICK-PREP, UNDER 20 MINUTES

Bacon and cheese for breakfast? Yes please! This simple breakfast recipe is delicious and portable. Just wrap it in aluminum foil and be on your way. Breakfast wraps are also versatile, so try using other ingredients like scallions, sour cream, scrambled eggs, mashed sweet potato, cubed tofu, thinly sliced red bell peppers, and more.

1 slice bacon

1 (6½-inch) soft corn tortilla

2 tablespoons shredded cheddar or Monterey Jack cheese

2 tablespoons mashed avocado

Sea salt

Freshly ground black pepper

½ teaspoon sriracha (optional)

1. Take the bacon out of the refrigerator 15 to 20 minutes before cooking. Lay the bacon on a cold skillet (don't preheat). Cook over medium heat and turn the slice as needed until it becomes crispy, 8 to 12 minutes. Drain well on a paper towel, then chop on a cutting board.

2. Set a medium skillet over medium-low heat. Put the tortilla in the skillet and top with the cheese and bacon. Warm until the cheese melts, 1 to 2 minutes.

3. Top with the mashed avocado and season with salt and pepper. Add the sriracha (if using).

FODMAP tip: *Up to 1 teaspoon of sriracha is low-FODMAP.*

Make-ahead tip: Cook 5 or more slices of bacon to use later for the Bacon Pecan Quinoa Salad (page 48), for breakfast, on a sandwich, or in another salad.

Substitution tip: Add scrambled eggs or firm tofu for extra protein.

Per serving: Calories: 269; Total fat: 19g; Total carbs: 14g; Fiber: 4g; Sugar: 0g; Protein: 12g; Sodium: 761mg

Breakfast Berry Parfait

Prep time: 2 minutes / Serves: 1

5 INGREDIENTS OR LESS, NUT-FREE, VEGETARIAN, QUICK-PREP, UNDER 10 MINUTES

Low-FODMAP plain lactose-free yogurt doesn't always have to be consumed alone or with fruit. This light and airy breakfast berry parfait can be dressed up so you can try something different for your morning meal or snack. One sweet taste and you'll feel like you're eating dessert for breakfast!

¼ **cup whipping cream**

¼ **cup heaped fresh blueberries**

1 **(6-ounce) tub lactose-free plain or vanilla yogurt**

⅛ **teaspoon granulated sugar**

½ **teaspoon lemon rind**

1. Pour the whipping cream into a glass measuring cup. With an electric mixer, whip the cream into soft peaks, 6 to 7 minutes. Set aside.

2. Drop the blueberries into a small parfait glass or glass cup. Fold in the yogurt and spread evenly over the blueberries.

3. Add dollops of the whipped cream, sprinkle with the sugar, and top with the lemon rind. Serve.

FODMAP tip: *Stick to plain or vanilla lactose-free yogurt for this recipe and don't use yogurt that already contains fruit as this recipe already contains a full serving of fruit.*

Per serving: Calories: 310; Total fat: 24g; Total carbs: 16g; Fiber: 1g; Sugar: 13g; Protein: 8g; Sodium: 102mg

Sweet Potato and Nut Breakfast Bowl

Prep time: 2 minutes / **Cook time:** 15 minutes / **Serves:** 1

VEGETARIAN, QUICK-PREP, UNDER 20 MINUTES

You can relish this wholesome breakfast bowl any day your gut desires it. It doesn't take much time to prepare this warm, filling recipe, and it also works well if you make it the night before to enjoy the next day. If you don't have pecans, you can opt to use a serving of another low-FODMAP nut.

1 medium sweet potato

¼ cup almond milk

½ cup cooked quinoa

1 tablespoon no-sugar-added dried cranberries

1 tablespoon butter (or vegan butter)

¼ teaspoon ground cinnamon

1 teaspoon maple syrup

⅛ teaspoon kosher salt

10 pecan halves or Candied Pecans (page 111)

1. Microwave the sweet potato for 4 minutes. Flip the potato and cook for another 3 minutes. If the potato isn't soft all the way through, cook for another 1 to 2 minutes.

2. Remove the sweet potato with tongs or a towel. Cut the potato in half and mash well with a fork. Scoop out the sweet potato and fill a measuring cup with ½ cup of mashed sweet potato. Put it in a small saucepot.

3. To the saucepot, add the almond milk, quinoa, cranberries, butter, cinnamon, maple syrup, and salt. Use a heavy spoon and stir to combine. Cook for 3 to 5 minutes, stirring every 30 seconds, until warmed through.

4. Transfer the sweet potato mixture to a bowl and top with the pecans. Serve warm.

FODMAP tip: *Only ½ cup of sweet potato is low-FODMAP. Anything higher becomes moderate- to high-FODMAP.*

Per serving: Calories: 452; Total fat: 29g; Total carbs: 44g; Fiber: 8g; Sugar: 10g; Protein: 8g; Sodium: 342mg

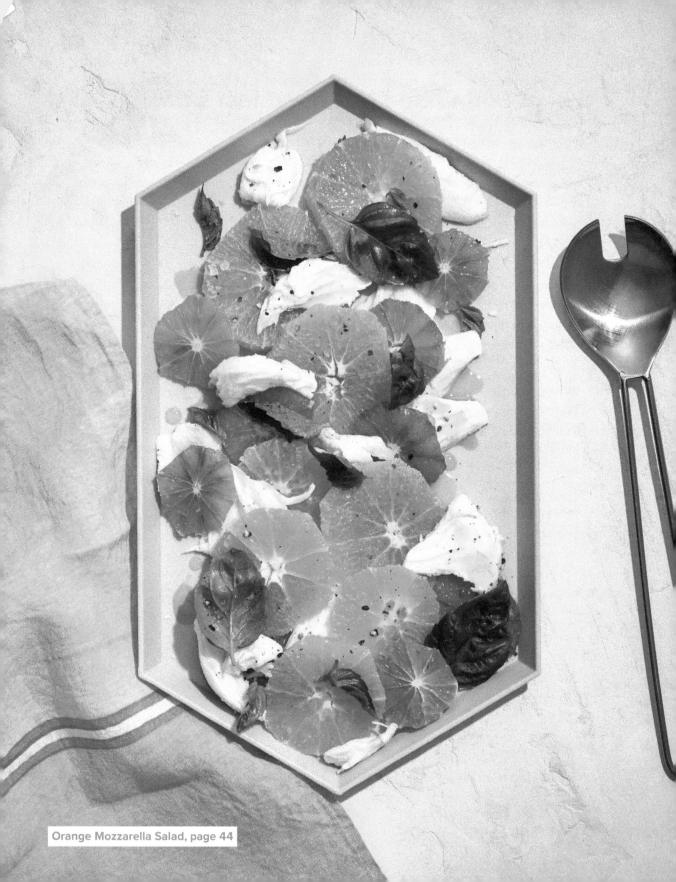

Orange Mozzarella Salad, page 44

CHAPTER 3

Sides and Salads

Quinoa Spinach

Prep time: 2 minutes / Cook time: 20 minutes / Serves: 8

DAIRY-FREE, NUT-FREE, QUICK-PREP, UNDER 30 MINUTES

This basic side dish is wonderful as is or dressed up with lemon juice, feta cheese, or chopped walnuts. There are several hacks for flavoring your foods while on the low-FODMAP diet—one is subbing out water for low-FODMAP broth when cooking quinoa, millet, polenta, or rice.

1 cup uncooked quinoa

1 tablespoon Garlic-Infused Oil (page 134)

2 cups low-FODMAP chicken broth

4 cups fresh baby spinach, packed, coarsely chopped

Kosher salt

Freshly ground black pepper

1. Rinse the quinoa in a fine wire mesh sieve under cold running water until the water runs clear; shake off any excess liquid.

2. Heat the oil in a large nonstick skillet over medium-high heat. Add the quinoa and cook, stirring frequently, until the quinoa starts to turn golden brown, about 2 minutes.

3. Add the broth to the skillet; bring to a boil. Cover the skillet and reduce the heat to low; simmer for 13 minutes. Stir in the spinach, cover the skillet, and cook until the spinach and quinoa are tender and the liquid is absorbed, about 3 to 5 minutes. Season with salt and pepper.

Ingredient tip: Casa de Sante makes a certified low-FODMAP Vegetable Stock Powder that would work perfectly for this recipe. All you have to do is add 2 teaspoons of the powder to 2 cups of hot water.

Per serving: Calories: 100; Total fat: 3g; Total carbs: 14g; Fiber: 2g; Sugar: 0g; Protein: 4g; Sodium: 30mg

Roasted Carrots with Macadamia Nuts and Tahini Dressing

Prep time: 2 minutes / **Cook time:** 25 minutes / **Serves:** 12

VEGAN, QUICK-PREP

This recipe is great any time of the year: Enjoy it during cold months indoors, during the holidays, or for celebrations outside. The carrots and dressing are so easy to make, and you'll love the way the ingredients complement each other. I like to pair this dish with poultry or baked tofu.

12 carrots

3 tablespoons Garlic-Infused Oil (page 134)

1¼ teaspoons kosher salt

½ teaspoon freshly ground black pepper

½ cup unsalted macadamia nuts

Tahini Dressing (page 139)

2 tablespoons minced fresh mint

1. Preheat the oven to 400°F. Line a baking sheet with parchment paper.

2. Cut the carrots on a diagonal and in thirds. Put them in a large bowl with the oil, salt, and pepper. Toss to coat. Transfer the carrots in an even layer to one side of the prepared baking sheet.

3. In the same large bowl, toss the macadamia nuts to coat them with the remaining oil mixture. Transfer the macadamia nuts to the other side of the baking sheet. Set the baking sheet on the top rack of the oven. Bake for 10 minutes, then put the macadamia nuts in a serving bowl. Continue baking the carrots for another 15 minutes or until tender.

4. In the serving bowl, toss the carrots with the dressing, mint, and macadamia nuts and serve.

Make-ahead tip: Make the Tahini Dressing ahead of time, and make extra to use on a salad or on other roasted low-FODMAP vegetables.

Per serving: Calories: 134; Total fat: 12g; Total carbs: 8g; Fiber: 2g; Sugar: 3g; Protein: 1g; Sodium: 257mg

Ⓕ Roasted Eggplant with Creamy Miso Sauce

Prep time: 10 minutes / Cook time: 20 minutes / Serves: 9

DAIRY-FREE, VEGETARIAN, UNDER 30 MINUTES

Use this recipe as an appetizer, a side dish with salmon, or in a sandwich with mozzarella cheese. Try my Creamy Miso Sauce on shrimp, lobster, in pasta, in a bowl with tofu, spread on sandwiches, on roasted vegetables, and more.

1½ pounds eggplant, cut into ½-inch rounds

2 tablespoons Garlic Infused Oil (page 134)

⅓ cup white miso

1 tablespoon grated fresh ginger

1 tablespoon sesame oil

1 teaspoon soy sauce

1 tablespoon maple syrup

1 tablespoon water

2 teaspoons rice vinegar

1 teaspoon sriracha

1 tablespoon sesame seeds

1. Preheat the oven to 450°F. Line a baking sheet with parchment paper.

2. Put the eggplant slices on the baking sheet, and lightly brush both sides of each round with the garlic infused oil. Bake until tender, about 18 minutes.

3. While the eggplant is baking, prepare the miso sauce and sesame seeds: In a small bowl, whisk together the miso, ginger, sesame oil, soy sauce, maple syrup, water, vinegar, and sriracha. Whisk until smooth. Heat the sesame seeds in a nonstick skillet over medium-low heat. Cook, stirring occasionally, until fragrant, about 8 minutes.

4. Remove the eggplant from the oven. Increase the oven temperature to broil.

5. Spread 1 to 2 teaspoons of miso sauce on each eggplant round (or just enough sauce to cover the tops). Put them in the oven and broil until browned, about 4 minutes. Sprinkle with the toasted sesame seeds.

FODMAP tip: *You can have up to 1 cup of eggplant per serving.*

Substitution tip: If you follow a gluten-free diet, you can use tamari instead of soy sauce.

Per serving: Calories: 94; Total fat: 6g; Total carbs: 9g; Fiber: 3g; Sugar: 4g; Protein: 2g; Sodium: 346mg

Curry Lentil and Spinach Soup

Prep time: 2 minutes / **Cook time:** 10 minutes / **Serves:** 4

NUT-FREE, VEGAN, QUICK-PREP, UNDER 20 MINUTES

Growing up, my mother, Rita, loved making me lentil soup with spinach and carrots. I've taken her recipe and transformed it into a sweet and spicy adventure for the senses. I can't eat as many lentils as I used to, but one serving of this soup is safe, low-FODMAP, and still reminds me of my mother's recipe.

1 tablespoon olive oil

1 medium carrot, peeled and thinly sliced

1 tablespoon curry powder

¼ teaspoon ground turmeric

1½ tablespoons finely grated fresh ginger

¼ teaspoon red pepper flakes

¾ cup canned lentils, drained and rinsed

1 (14.5-ounce) can crushed tomatoes

¾ cup canned unsweetened coconut milk

3 teaspoons packed brown sugar

2 cups baby spinach, loosely packed

¼ cup chopped cilantro

¼ teaspoon kosher salt

2 cups low-FODMAP vegetable broth

¼ teaspoon or more freshly ground black pepper

1. Heat the oil in a medium saucepan over medium heat. Add the carrot and cook for 2 minutes. Add the curry powder, turmeric, ginger, and red pepper flakes and stir constantly for 30 seconds.

2. Drain and rinse the lentils with water over a strainer. Add the lentils to the saucepan along with the tomatoes, coconut milk, sugar, spinach, cilantro, and salt and stir to combine; cook for 2 minutes.

3. Slowly add the low-FODMAP broth to the saucepan, stir again to combine; season with pepper. Turn the heat up to medium-high and cook for 5 minutes. Serve hot.

FODMAP tip: *Make sure when you buy curry powder that it does not contain onion, garlic, or "spices," which could also be onion or garlic. For canned lentils, stick to ½ cup per serving.*

Per serving: Calories: 248; Total fat: 15g; Total carbs: 26g; Fiber: 7g; Sugar: 6g; Protein: 7g; Sodium: 397mg

Orange Mozzarella Salad

Prep time: 5 minutes / Serves: 4

NUT-FREE, VEGETARIAN, QUICK-PREP, UNDER 10 MINUTES

This orange mozzarella salad is simple but has a lot of flavor! You will love the velvety taste of mozzarella and olive oil paired with the navel oranges and basil. Since you need to stick to one serving of low-FODMAP fruit for every meal, limit yourself to two servings of this salad.

2 medium navel oranges, peeled

5 ounces fresh mozzarella cheese, diced

½ ounce fresh basil leaves, chopped

1 tablespoon extra-virgin olive oil

⅛ teaspoon kosher salt, plus more for seasoning

⅛ teaspoon freshly ground black pepper

1. Cut the oranges into 1-inch wheels and put them in a serving bowl.

2. Add the mozzarella and chop the basil.

3. Add the olive oil, salt, and pepper to the serving bowl. Toss to combine and add more salt if desired. Serve.

Serving tip: If you're going to make this salad ahead of time, be sure to leave the salad out for a few minutes before serving so the oil can warm to room temperature.

Per serving: Calories: 159; Total fat: 10g; Total carbs: 8g; Fiber: 2g; Sugar: 6g; Protein: 7g; Sodium: 130mg

Crunchy Asian-Inspired Salad

Prep time: 10 minutes / **Serves:** 8

VEGAN, UNDER 20 MINUTES

This salad goes very well with my Asian-Style Fusion Salmon (page 78) and can be dressed up with my Asian-Style Salad Dressing (page 142). All the raw ingredients make this a very crunchy and refreshing salad.

4 cups chopped
   green cabbage

3 cups chopped
   butter lettuce

3 scallions, green parts
   only, chopped

⅓ cup fresh
   cilantro, chopped

⅓ medium celery
   stalk, finely diced

1 medium carrot,
   peeled and grated

1 cup shelled frozen
   edamame, thawed

3 tablespoons chopped
   peanuts (roasted
   if possible)

1 tablespoon sesame seeds

In a large salad serving bowl, combine the cabbage, lettuce, scallions, cilantro, and celery and toss. Add the carrot and edamame. Toss together with the chopped peanuts and sesame seeds. Serve with dressing.

FODMAP tip: *Celery is low-FODMAP at 10 grams per serving. The amount of celery in this recipe is very little per serving as it is spread across eight servings.*

Per serving: Calories: 77; Total fat: 4g; Total carbs: 8g; Fiber: 3g; Sugar: 2g; Protein: 6g; Sodium: 19mg

Radish, Fennel, and Butter Beans Salad

Prep time: 4 minutes / Serves: 1

VEGAN, QUICK-PREP, UNDER 10 MINUTES

This hybrid salad is perfect for winter or summer. Fennel is low-FODMAP as long as only the bulb is used. The butter beans make a great addition and provide protein, B vitamins, iron, and fiber. This salad tastes best when covered and refrigerated for up to one hour before serving.

¼ **cup canned butter beans, drained and rinsed**

¼ **cup fresh parsley leaves, chopped**

1 radish, very thinly sliced

½ **cup very thinly sliced fennel bulb**

½ **cup baby arugula**

½ **teaspoon drained capers**

Lemon zest from ½ **medium lemon**

1 teaspoon freshly squeezed lemon juice, plus more as needed

1 tablespoon extra-virgin olive oil

⅛ **teaspoon kosher salt**

¼ **teaspoon freshly ground black pepper**

1. In a medium bowl, combine the butter beans, parsley, radish, fennel, arugula, and capers.

2. In a small bowl, combine the lemon zest, lemon juice, olive oil, salt, and pepper. Stir or whisk to combine and pour over the salad. Toss the salad and serve.

FODMAP tip: A ½-cup of fennel bulb is equal to one low-FODMAP serving. Anything more becomes moderate- to high-FODMAP. A ¼-cup of canned butter beans is equal to one low-FODMAP serving. Anything more becomes moderate- to high-FODMAP.

Per serving: Calories: 185; Total fat: 15g; Total carbs: 12g; Fiber: 4g; Sugar: 1g; Protein: 4g; Sodium: 72mg

Warm Kale, Pine Nut, and Pomegranate Salad

Prep time: 2 minutes / Cook time: 10 minutes / Serves: 4

VEGETARIAN, QUICK-PREP, UNDER 10 MINUTES

The season for pomegranate seeds typically runs from October through February, but many grocers carry pomegranate seeds all year long. As long as you have access to these red, juicy seeds, this is another salad that could work well any time of year.

2 teaspoons freshly squeezed lemon juice

⅛ teaspoon kosher salt

¼ teaspoon freshly ground black pepper

2 tablespoons extra-virgin olive oil

¼ cup pine nuts

3½ ounces baby kale

Cooking oil spray

4 tablespoons shaved Parmesan cheese, divided

½ cup pomegranate seeds

1. In a medium serving bowl, whisk the lemon juice, salt, pepper, and oil.

2. Put the pine nuts in a small dry sauté pan or skillet and cook for 3 minutes over medium heat, stirring frequently until golden. Remove from the heat.

3. Prepare the kale by cutting out the ribs and slicing ribbons from the green leaves. Add the kale to a medium pan lightly sprayed with oil. Sauté until the kale is deep green but not yet wilted, 4 to 5 minutes.

4. To the large bowl, add the kale, Parmesan cheese, and pine nuts; toss to combine. Sprinkle the pomegranate seeds on top and serve.

FODMAP tip: *One low-FODMAP serving of pomegranate seeds is 45 grams.*

Per serving: Calories: 167; Total fat: 14g; Total carbs: 8g; Fiber: 1g; Sugar: 2g; Protein: 4g; Sodium: 116mg

Ⓕ Bacon Pecan Quinoa Salad

Prep time: 5 minutes / Cook time: 28 minutes, plus 5 minutes for the quinoa to rest / Serves: 2

QUICK-PREP

When paired with Maple Vinaigrette, this salad is sweet, salty, and very satisfying. Preparing the quinoa and bacon ahead of time makes this recipe very easy to pull together.

1 cup uncooked quinoa

2 cups water

Pinch salt

4 slices bacon

Maple Vinaigrette (page 137)

4 cups baby spinach, chopped

10 cherry tomatoes, halved

10 pecan halves or Candied Pecans (page 111), optional

1. Rinse the quinoa in a fine mesh sieve until the water runs clear, then drain and transfer to a medium pot. Add the water and salt and bring to a boil. Cover, reduce the heat to medium-low, and simmer until the water is absorbed, 15 to 20 minutes. Remove from the heat for 5 minutes; uncover and fluff with a fork. Transfer the quinoa to a serving bowl.

2. Lay the bacon slices on a cold skillet (don't preheat). Cook over medium heat and turn the slices as needed until they become crispy, about 8 minutes. Drain well on a paper towel, then chop on a cutting board.

3. While the bacon is cooking, make the maple vinaigrette.

4. Transfer the chopped bacon to a serving bowl, followed by the spinach, tomatoes, and pecans (if using). Toss to combine and drizzle in 2 to 4 tablespoons of the maple vinaigrette. Serve.

FODMAP tip: *One low-FODMAP serving of cherry tomatoes is equal to about 5 cherry tomatoes.*

Per serving: Calories: 765; Total fat: 40g; Total carbs: 71g; Fiber: 10g; Sugar: 9g; Protein: 30g; Sodium: 1161mg

Taco Chopped Salad

Prep time: 2 minutes / Cook time: 15 minutes / Serves: 4

NUT-FREE, QUICK-PREP, UNDER 20 MINUTES

This tasty salad is great for lunch and keeps well in the refrigerator for a couple of days. Most taco salads contain high-FODMAP ingredients. I've included low-FODMAP alternatives (such as chickpeas instead of beans) as well as a recipe in the tips section to make taco seasoning at home.

1 pound lean ground beef

½ cup canned chickpeas, drained and rinsed

½ tablespoon Fody Foods™ Low FODMAP Taco Seasoning

⅔ cup water

1 head iceberg lettuce, chopped (about 8 cups)

1 cup shredded cheddar cheese

1 small tomato, chopped

2 tablespoons chopped fresh cilantro

2 cups corn chips or corn tortilla chips

4 tablespoons low-FODMAP ranch dressing

1 medium lime, quartered

1. In a large skillet, cook the beef over medium heat for 6 to 8 minutes, until no longer pink; drain. Stir in the chickpeas, taco seasoning, and water; bring to a boil. Reduce the heat; simmer, uncovered, 3 to 4 minutes or until thickened, stirring occasionally.

2. In 4 separate bowls, layer the lettuce, cheese, beef mixture, tomato, and cilantro. Serve with chips and add 1 tablespoon of dressing to each salad along with a wedge of lime.

FODMAP tip: *A ¼-cup serving of canned chickpeas is low-FODMAP. Always remember to drain and rinse the chickpeas before consuming.*

Ingredient tip: Make your own taco seasoning by combining 1 tablespoon chili powder, ¼ teaspoon red pepper flakes, a dash of wheat-free asafetida powder, ½ teaspoon dried oregano, ½ teaspoon paprika, 1½ teaspoons ground cumin, 1 teaspoon sea salt, and 1 teaspoon freshly ground black pepper. Save unused seasoning in an airtight container.

Substitution tip: If you do not have certified low-FODMAP ranch dressing, 1 tablespoon of lactose-free sour cream is a great substitute.

Per serving: Calories: 508; Total fat: 31g; Total carbs: 26g; Fiber: 3g; Sugar: 3g; Protein: 33g; Sodium: 762mg

Colorful Crunchy Salad

Prep time: 15 minutes / Serves: 4

NUT-FREE, VEGAN, UNDER 20 MINUTES

This super colorful, crunchy, and healthy salad is very filling and tastes divine with Carrot Ginger Dressing. I like serving this salad along with grilled salmon, shredded chicken, or pork.

6 ounces chopped butter lettuce or romaine

1 cup frozen edamame, defrosted

1 cup chopped common cabbage

¾ cup finely sliced broccoli heads

½ medium red bell pepper, chopped

⅓ cup roughly chopped fresh cilantro

1 tablespoon chopped scallions, white parts only

Carrot Ginger Dressing (page 138)

1. In a large serving bowl, combine the lettuce, edamame, cabbage, broccoli, red bell pepper, cilantro, and scallions.

2. Add 2 to 4 tablespoons of dressing and toss to lightly coat all the ingredients.

Storage tip: Store the leftover salad separately from the dressing, and toss individual servings with dressing just before serving. The salad will keep for 3 to 4 days in the refrigerator.

Per serving: Calories: 146; Total fat: 9g; Total carbs: 16g; Fiber: 5g; Sugar: 6g; Protein: 10g; Sodium: 29mg

Eggplant Pasta Salad

Prep time: 5 minutes / **Cook time:** 20 minutes, plus 30 minutes to sit / **Serves:** 4

NUT-FREE, VEGETARIAN

Warm eggplant, pasta, and melted cheese make this a very appetizing dish for lunch or dinner, or for your next social gathering. Eggplant is low-FODMAP at 1 cup per serving and has about 2.5 grams of fiber.

1 medium eggplant, cut into 1-inch slices and then quartered

¼ teaspoon kosher salt, plus more for salting eggplant

1 teaspoon Garlic-Infused Oil (page 134)

1½ tablespoons red wine vinegar

½ teaspoon freshly ground black pepper

¼ teaspoon red pepper flakes

¼ teaspoon dried thyme leaves

¼ teaspoon dried oregano

10 ounces gluten-free penne pasta

1 tablespoon vegetable oil

20 to 30 cherry tomatoes

8 ounces fresh mozzarella, cut into cubes

1 cup fresh basil leaves

1. Put the eggplant pieces in a colander and toss with salt. Allow to sit for 20 to 30 minutes.

2. In a large serving bowl, whisk together the oil, red wine vinegar, the remaining ¼ teaspoon of salt, pepper, red pepper flakes, thyme, and oregano.

3. Cook the pasta according to the package directions.

4. While the pasta is cooking, heat the vegetable oil in a skillet over medium-high heat. Cook the eggplant for 6 to 8 minutes, then flip each piece. Add the cherry tomatoes. Wait 5 minutes before tossing.

5. After 3 minutes, toss the mixture again. The eggplant and tomatoes should be slightly charred, with the tomatoes slightly bursting. Transfer the mixture to a serving bowl.

6. Drain the pasta and immediately add it to the bowl with the vegetables. Add the cheese and toss gently to combine. Top with the basil and serve immediately.

FODMAP tip: *Different types of cherry tomatoes vary in weight. Depending on the type of cherry tomatoes you choose, you can add up to 300 grams for this recipe. Make sure the gluten-free pasta is low FODMAP (i.e. no legume flour [besan, chickpea, soy, or urid]).*

Per serving: Calories: 429; Total fat: 15g; Total carbs: 57g; Fiber: 6g; Sugar: 4g; Protein: 16g; Sodium: 294mg

Collard Greens and Pancetta

Prep time: 5 minutes / Cook time: 20 minutes / Serves: 2

DAIRY-FREE, NUT-FREE, QUICK-PREP, UNDER 30 MINUTES

This lovely side dish can be made into a meal by mixing it with 2 servings of warm pasta and topping it with Parmesan cheese. Pancetta is flavorful and low-FODMAP, but stick to the serving size noted in this recipe, as foods that are higher in fat can become gut irritants.

1 bunch fresh collard greens (to yield 4 cups)

3 tablespoons pancetta

½ tablespoon Garlic Infused Oil (page 134)

¾ cup low-FODMAP chicken broth, divided

1 teaspoon freshly squeezed lemon juice

⅛ teaspoon sea salt

⅛ teaspoon freshly ground black pepper

¼ teaspoon red pepper flakes (optional)

1. Prepare the collard greens. Run a knife along the ribs and cut them out, then slice the greens into ribbons.

2. In a large skillet, fry the pancetta in the oil over medium-low heat, until the solid fat is melted, rendering it from the meat.

3. Add the collard greens and ¼ cup of broth. Simmer gently until the broth evaporates, about 2 minutes, then add another ¼ cup. Wait until the liquid evaporates again and add the last ¼ cup of broth. Add the lemon juice. Season with salt and pepper and sprinkle with red pepper flakes (if using). Serve.

Ingredient tip: Use my Vegetable Herb Broth (page 128) or Chicken Stock (page 129).

Per serving: Calories: 173; Total fat: 13g; Total carbs: 6g; Fiber: 3g; Sugar: 0g; Protein: 11g; Sodium: 758mg

Creamy Mediterranean Pasta Salad

Prep time: 5 minutes / **Cook time:** 15 minutes / **Serves:** 5

NUT-FREE, VEGETARIAN, QUICK-PREP, UNDER 30 MINUTES

This creamy pasta salad is full of fresh Mediterranean flavor and pairs well with lean meat or fish. Although there are a few ingredients required, it's fast to make and full of flavor.

1 (6-ounce) container low-fat plain Greek yogurt

⅓ cup mayonnaise

5 ounces feta cheese crumbles

1 teaspoon red wine vinegar

1 teaspoon freshly squeezed lemon juice

1½ tablespoons kosher salt plus ¼ teaspoon, divided

¼ teaspoon freshly ground black pepper, divided, plus more for seasoning

2½ tablespoons Garlic-Infused Oil (page 134), divided

8 ounces gluten-free fusilli

12 pitted green olives, chopped

¼ teaspoon dried oregano

1 tablespoon chopped fresh chives

2 tablespoons roughly chopped fresh basil

2 tablespoons roughly chopped fresh flat-leaf parsley

20 cherry tomatoes, halved

5 cups baby spinach (optional)

1. In a medium bowl, mix together the yogurt, mayonnaise, feta cheese, red wine vinegar, lemon juice, salt, black pepper, and 2 tablespoons of oil. Set aside.

2. Fill a medium pot three-quarters full with cold water, bring to a boil, and add 1½ tablespoons of salt. Add the fusilli and cook until al dente, 8 to 10 minutes. The pasta should be firm when bitten with a slightly dense center and softer outside. Drain, transfer the pasta to a large bowl, and mix with about ½ tablespoon of oil.

3. To the large bowl with the warm fusilli, add the olives, oregano, chives, basil, parsley, and additional pepper (if desired). Add the dressing and mix well with a rubber spatula to combine. Add the cherry tomatoes and mix gently again. Serve atop the baby spinach (if using).

FODMAP tip: *Make sure the Greek yogurt is strained. Straining helps lower the lactose content, making a 6-ounce serving or less low-FODMAP.*

Per serving: Calories: 500; Total fat: 22g; Total carbs: 64g; Fiber: 5g; Sugar: 4g; Protein: 16g; Sodium: 577mg

Warm Chicken Salad with Greens and Pumpkin Seeds

Prep time: 2 minutes / Cook time: 25 minutes / Serves: 2

NUT-FREE, QUICK-PREP, UNDER 30 MINUTES

This warm and filling salad is full of protein and flavor. Many healthy, low-FODMAP, and nutrient-dense ingredients are included. Quinoa is a healthy low-FODMAP protein that includes nine essential amino acids.

½ **teaspoon kosher salt**

1 **bay leaf**

1 **pound boneless, skinless chicken breast**

1 **endive**

2 **cups chopped butter lettuce**

1 **cup arugula**

⅓ **cup fresh basil, chopped**

⅓ **cup fresh cilantro, chopped**

1 **cup chopped green cabbage**

2 **tablespoons pumpkin seeds**

1 **tablespoon cold water**

½ **cup cooked quinoa**

1 **navel orange, peeled and cut into quarters**

2 **ounces goat cheese (optional)**

1. Fill a pot with 1½ inches of cold water, salt, and the bay leaf. Place the chicken breast in an even layer on the bottom of the pot and heat over medium heat until the water just barely begins to simmer, then reduce the heat to low and cook for 15 minutes. The chicken breasts will be done once they are no longer pink in the middle or the internal temperature has reached 165°F.

2. While the chicken is cooking, trim the stem ends off the endive and cut lengthwise down the center. Cut out the core from the center of the endive and pull the leaves apart.

3. Assemble your salad in a large serving bowl. Combine the endive, lettuce, arugula, basil, cilantro, cabbage, and pumpkin seeds. Toss to combine.

4. Reheat the quinoa by placing it in a bowl with the cold water. Cover the bowl with a paper towel and cook in the microwave for 1 minute. Add the quinoa to the serving bowl.

5. Once the chicken is done, put it on a cutting board, and pat away any excess water with a paper towel. Slice the breasts horizontally, creating thin pieces.

6. Add the chicken and orange to the salad. Mix well to combine and add the goat cheese (if using). Serve immediately with your low-FODMAP dressing of choice.

Per serving: Calories: 446; Total fat: 11g; Total carbs: 31g; Fiber: 6g; Sugar: 11g; Protein: 55g; Sodium: 283mg

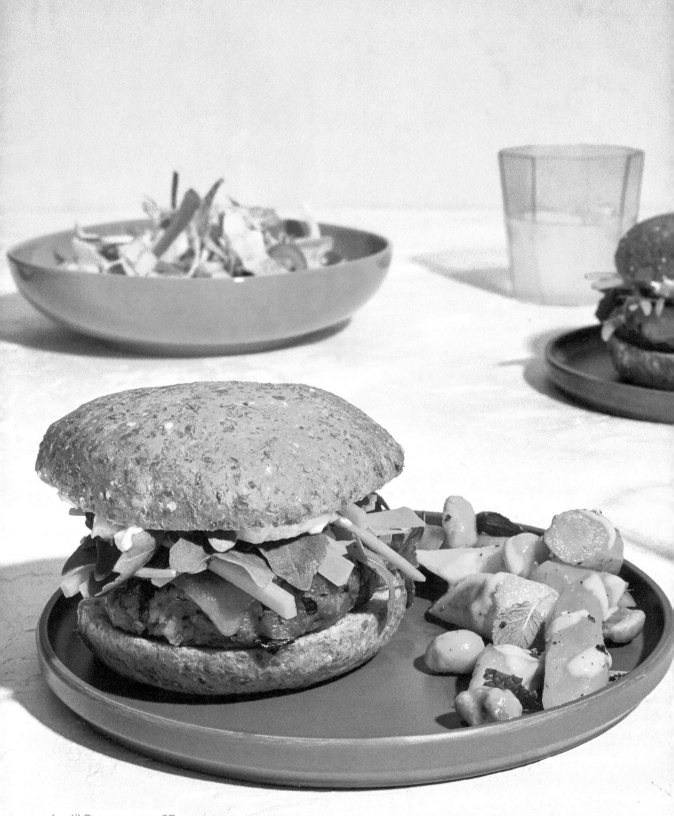

Lentil Burgers, page 67

CHAPTER 4

Meatless Mains

Green Tea Goddess Risotto

Prep time: 5 minutes / Cook time: 30 minutes / Serves: 4

ONE POT, VEGAN, QUICK-PREP

This creamy, dairy-free risotto marries well with the herbaceous flavors of the green goddess dressing. Brewed green tea leaves add new layers of complexity to this classic comfort food.

5 cups water

6 green tea bags

2 tablespoons sesame oil

1 tablespoon Casa de Sante Low-FODMAP Certified Vegetable Stock Powder

1 teaspoon ground ginger

1½ cups sushi rice

1 cup fresh parsley

¼ cup thinly sliced scallions (green parts only)

3 cups fresh arugula, divided

¼ cup pine nuts

⅓ cup freshly squeezed lemon juice

1½ cups shelled edamame

1 teaspoon kosher salt

1. Put the water and green tea in a medium saucepan over medium heat and cover with a lid. Bring to a boil, turn off the heat, and let steep for 5 minutes. Remove the tea bags, setting 3 aside.

2. Stir in the sesame oil, stock powder, ginger, and rice and bring the tea mixture back to a boil. Reduce the heat to medium-low, cover, and let simmer gently for 18 to 22 minutes, until the grains are tender and creamy. When fully cooked, the rice should be neither dry nor soupy.

3. Meanwhile, put the parsley, scallions, and 2 cups of arugula in a food processor. Open the reserved tea bags, add the green tea leaves, and pulse. Add the pine nuts and slowly drizzle the lemon juice while pulsing, until the mixture is coarsely ground like pesto.

4. Fold the herb mixture into the risotto along with the edamame and salt. Stir until thoroughly incorporated.

5. Divide equally between 4 bowls, top each with the remaining 1 cup of arugula, and serve.

Storage tip: Store leftover risotto in an airtight container in the refrigerator for 2 to 3 days. Reheat in a medium saucepan over medium-low heat along with an additional splash of water. Stir periodically until hot all the way through, 4 to 6 minutes.

Per serving: Calories: 440; Total fat: 16g; Total carbs: 63g; Fiber: 5g; Sugar: 3g; Protein: 13g; Sodium: 163mg

Palak Tofu

Prep time: 10 minutes / **Cook time:** 30 minutes / **Serves:** 4

NUT-FREE, VEGAN

Silky simmered spinach meets exotic Indian spices in this bold green entrée. Lightly baked cubes of tofu replace the traditional paneer for a lower-fat, higher-protein entrée. Serve with basmati rice to soak up all that luscious, spicy sauce.

14 ounces firm tofu, cut into 1-inch cubes

¼ cup Shallot-Infused Oil (page 136), divided

2 tablespoons freshly squeezed lemon juice

1 teaspoon kosher salt, divided

1 tablespoon minced fresh ginger

1 jalapeño pepper, seeded and minced

1 tablespoon whole coriander seeds

2 teaspoons whole cumin seeds

½ teaspoon ground turmeric

¼ teaspoon ground cardamom

¼ teaspoon cayenne pepper

¼ teaspoon asafetida (optional)

½ cup water

1 pound (about 12 cups) fresh baby spinach

2 cups cooked basmati rice, to serve

1. Preheat the oven to 375°F. Toss the tofu with 2 tablespoons of oil, lemon juice, and ½ teaspoon of salt in a small baking dish. Spread the pieces out in an even layer and bake for 20 minutes until lightly golden brown around the edges. Set aside.

2. Meanwhile, heat the remaining oil in a 14-inch pot over medium-high heat. Add the ginger and jalapeño pepper and cook for 2 to 3 minutes, until aromatic. Mix in the coriander, cumin, turmeric, cardamom, cayenne, and asafetida (if using), stirring constantly for 2 minutes.

3. Quickly pour in the water to prevent the spices from over-toasting or burning. Bring to a gentle simmer.

4. Add the spinach a few handfuls at a time, stirring gently until it wilts. Season with the remaining ½ teaspoon of salt. This process should take about 10 minutes.

5. Transfer the spinach mixture to a blender or food processor and blend for about 1 minute to create a coarse stew. Unlike a smooth purée, it should still have a good amount of texture to it.

6. Return the purée to the stove, along with the baked tofu. Simmer over medium heat for 5 to 10 minutes until warmed through.

7. Serve immediately over the hot basmati rice.

Storage tip: Store leftovers in an airtight container in the refrigerator for up to 3 days.

Per serving: Calories: 386; Total fat: 18g; Total carbs: 45g; Fiber: 5g; Sugar: 2g; Protein: 15g; Sodium: 228mg

Soba Noodle Lo Mein

Prep time: 5 minutes / Cook time: 20 minutes / Serves: 4

NUT-FREE, ONE POT, VEGAN, QUICK-PREP, UNDER 30 MINUTES

Quicker than ordering delivery, this wholesome take on the takeout classic satisfies in a flash. The soba noodles lend a hearty bite that's lightened with a generous serving of fresh, crisp vegetables. This might be your new busy weeknight go-to dinner!

9 ounces gluten-free soba noodles

2 tablespoons Garlic-Infused Oil (page 134), divided

8 ounces extra-firm tofu, cubed

1 red bell pepper, seeded and thinly sliced

1 cup shredded carrot

1 cup canned baby corn, cut in half lengthwise

½ cup sliced water chestnuts

2 cups sliced baby bok choy

1 cup canned champignon mushrooms, drained

2 tablespoons soy sauce, or more if desired

½ teaspoon ground ginger

2 tablespoons thinly sliced scallions (green parts only)

1. Bring a large saucepan or pot of water to a boil over medium heat and cook the soba noodles until just al dente, about 3 minutes. Drain and immediately rinse with cold water. Set aside.

2. Heat 1 tablespoon of oil in a wok or 12-inch skillet over high heat. Add the tofu and cook for 8 to 10 minutes, flipping carefully to keep the cubes intact, until brown on all sides. Transfer to a plate and set aside.

3. Coat the skillet or wok with the remaining 1 tablespoon of oil and return it to the stove over high heat. Sauté the bell pepper, carrot, corn, water chestnuts, and bok choy, stirring constantly. Stir-fry for 4 to 6 minutes until the vegetables are tender and aromatic.

4. Add the mushrooms, cooked soba noodles, and tofu. Mix together the soy sauce and ginger before pouring on top, tossing thoroughly to combine. Cook for 1 to 2 minutes longer.

5. Top with the sliced scallions and serve.

Storage tip: Store leftovers in an airtight container in the refrigerator for 2 to 3 days.

Per serving: Calories: 417; Total fat: 12g; Total carbs: 69g; Fiber: 3g; Sugar: 5g; Protein: 19g; Sodium: 1015mg

Spring Roll Bowl

Prep time: 5 minutes / Cook time: 25 minutes / Serves: 4

NUT-FREE OPTION, VEGAN

Skip the fuss and frustration of wrapping individual spring rolls. Tossing everything into large bowls lets you load up on more vegetables for a more satisfying meal. The combination of bright, fresh herbs makes this a refreshing choice on a hot summer day.

For the baked tofu

- 8 ounces extra-firm tofu, cut into ¼-inch rectangles
- 3 tablespoons soy sauce
- 1 tablespoon Fody™ garlic oil
- ½ teaspoon five spice powder

For the noodles and vegetables

- 8 ounces dried thin rice noodles (vermicelli)
- 1 seedless cucumber, peeled and thinly sliced
- 1 cup shredded carrots
- 1 red bell pepper, seeded and thinly sliced
- 1 cup bean sprouts
- 8 radishes, thinly sliced
- ¼ cup pineapple juice
- 2 tablespoons rice vinegar
- ¼ cup fresh mint, chopped
- ½ cup fresh basil, chopped
- ¼ cup peanuts, chopped (optional)

1. Preheat the oven to 400°F and arrange a single layer of sliced tofu in a 13-by-9-inch baking pan. Whisk together the soy sauce, oil, and five spice powder in a separate bowl before drizzling evenly over the tofu. Bake for 20 to 25 minutes, flipping halfway through, until golden brown on both sides.

2. Meanwhile, bring a large pot of water to a boil over high heat, add the noodles, and cook for 1 to 2 minutes until tender. Immediately drain and rinse under cold water.

3. Toss the cucumber, carrots, bell pepper, sprouts, and radishes in a large bowl, along with the cooked rice noodles, pineapple juice, and rice vinegar. Mix thoroughly to combine.

4. Divide between 4 bowls and top with equal amounts of the baked tofu, mint, basil, and chopped peanuts (if using).

Ingredient tip: Use brown rice noodles to add more fiber without sacrificing flavor. Depending on the thickness, they may take longer to cook than plain white rice noodles, so check the instructions on the packaging for the precise cook time.

Per serving: Calories: 391; Total fat: 11g; Total carbs: 62g; Fiber: 4g; Sugar: 6g; Protein: 12g; Sodium: 714mg

Tempeh Satay Sandwiches

Prep time: 10 minutes / Cook time: 20 minutes / Serves: 2

VEGAN

Just about anything would taste good coated in rich, spicy peanut sauce, but this hearty sandwich is especially delicious. Thick slabs of tempeh meet the satisfying crunch of fresh vegetables and toasted bread, dazzling in ways the average PB&J can only dream of.

For the satay sauce

3 tablespoons soy sauce

2 tablespoons rice vinegar

1 teaspoon minced fresh ginger

1 teaspoon Fody™ vegetable soup base

½ teaspoon red pepper flakes

2 drops liquid stevia (optional)

½ cup creamy peanut butter

¾ cup water

For the tempeh sandwich

1 tablespoon sesame oil

1 (8-ounce) package tempeh

4 slices sourdough bread, toasted

4 leaves romaine, red leaf, or butter lettuce

1 cup shredded carrots

2 medium tomatoes, sliced

1. In a large bowl, whisk together the soy sauce, rice vinegar, ginger, soup base, red pepper flakes, and stevia (if using). Stir in the peanut butter and slowly begin drizzling in the water. It will be very thick at first, but continue to add the liquid until the mixture is similar to the consistency of barbeque sauce.

2. In a large nonstick pan, heat the sesame oil over medium-high heat. Slice the tempeh into 2 equal squares. Put it in the pan, making sure the pieces don't overlap. Pour about 1 cup of satay sauce on top and bring to a gentle simmer. Cook for about 10 minutes before flipping. Continue to cook for another 10 minutes, until it's darkened around the edges and the sauce clings to both sides.

3. To assemble the sandwiches, top 2 slices of toasted bread with lettuce, carrots, sliced tomato, tempeh, and the final piece of bread.

Storage tip: To keep the sandwich from being too messy for a grab-and-go meal, wrap it tightly in parchment paper, cut it in half, and then rewrap it in aluminum foil. Store extra satay sauce in an airtight container in the refrigerator for up to 1 week.

Per serving: Calories: 916; Total fat: 53g; Total carbs: 73g; Fiber: 9g; Sugar: 14g; Protein: 48g; Sodium: 2120mg

Pasta with Broccoli and Bread Crumbs

Prep time: 5 minutes / Cook time: 15 minutes / Serves: 4

NUT-FREE, VEGETARIAN, QUICK-PREP, UNDER 30 MINUTES

I grew up with this comforting meal. The plain bread crumbs and Garlic-Infused Oil really bring in the taste of garlic without the pesky FODMAPs.

1 pound thin gluten-free spaghetti

3 cups broccoli florets

1 cup plain gluten-free bread crumbs

½ teaspoon dried oregano

¼ teaspoon dried thyme

½ cup Garlic-Infused Oil (page 134)

½ teaspoon red pepper flakes

½ cup shaved Parmesan cheese

1. Prepare the pasta according to the package directions.

2. While the pasta is cooking, add the broccoli to a pot of boiling water for a couple of minutes, then remove and immediately put it in cold water to stop the cooking. Set aside.

3. In a small bowl, combine the bread crumbs, oregano, and thyme. Mix and set aside.

4. In a large skillet, heat the oil. Add the red pepper flakes. Cook for 1 minute then add the bread crumb mixture. Stir constantly for 2 more minutes, until the bread crumbs become crunchy and golden.

5. Add the broccoli and stir for another minute.

6. Drain the pasta and add it to the skillet. Cook everything together for another minute. Serve immediately topped with Parmesan cheese.

Ingredient tip: Make sure the bread crumbs are gluten-free and don't contain high-FODMAP ingredients (see page 145 for some reliable brands).

Per serving: Calories: 754; Total fat: 31g; Total carbs: 99g; Fiber: 12g; Sugar: 3g; Protein: 20g; Sodium: 339mg

(F) Squash and Goat Cheese Brown Rice Bowl

Prep time: 3 minutes / Cook time: 30 minutes / Serves: 1

NUT-FREE, VEGETARIAN, QUICK-PREP

This satisfying bowl blends different flavors and textures with healthy nutri-ents to help you power through the day. Feel free to use quinoa instead of rice, substitute arugula for spinach, try a different low-FODMAP cheese, or throw in sunflower seeds, walnuts, or macadamia nuts.

⅓ **cup cubed butternut squash**

1 **tablespoon extra-virgin olive oil, divided**

¼ **teaspoon kosher salt, divided**

¼ **teaspoon freshly ground black pepper**

1 **tablespoon balsamic vinegar**

½ **teaspoon Dijon mustard**

½ **teaspoon honey**

¾ **cup cooked brown rice**

1 **cup fresh baby spinach**

1 **ounce soft goat cheese**

½ **tablespoon pumpkin seeds**

1. Preheat the oven to 400°F.

2. Toss the butternut squash with ½ tablespoon of olive oil in a bowl. Season with ⅛ teaspoon each of salt and pepper. Arrange the coated squash on a baking sheet.

3. Roast in the preheated oven until the squash is tender and lightly browned, about 25 minutes.

4. In a small bowl, whisk together the remaining ½ tablespoon of olive oil, the balsamic vinegar, Dijon mustard, honey, and the remaining ⅛ teaspoon of salt.

5. Add the cooked rice to a microwave-safe bowl and reheat for 1 to 2 minutes.

6. Add the butternut squash and spinach to the bowl of brown rice, and toss to combine. Top with the goat cheese, pumpkin seeds, and dressing.

FODMAP tip: A ⅓-cup roasted butternut squash is a low-FODMAP serving. Anything more becomes moderate- to high-FODMAP.

Per serving: Calories: 376; Total fat: 23g; Total carbs: 35g; Fiber: 3g; Sugar: 4g; Protein: 10g; Sodium: 199mg

Greek Quinoa Bowl

Prep time: 5 minutes / **Serves:** 1

NUT-FREE, VEGETARIAN, QUICK-PREP, UNDER 20 MINUTES

This healthy take on a Greek bowl is so easy to prepare, especially if you've prepared the quinoa ahead of time.

½ tablespoon
  extra-virgin olive oil

1 tablespoon
  balsamic vinegar

½ teaspoon stone-ground
  Dijon mustard

½ teaspoon honey

⅛ teaspoon kosher
  salt, plus more for
  seasoning (optional)

¾ cup cooked quinoa

1 teaspoon freshly
  squeezed lemon juice

5 cherry tomatoes, halved

8 black pitted olives

2 slices cucumber,
  cut into quarters

1 ounce feta cheese

Freshly ground black
  pepper (optional)

1. Whisk together the olive oil, balsamic vinegar, Dijon mustard, honey, and salt.

2. Place the quinoa in a serving bowl. Top with the lemon juice, tomatoes, olives, cucumber, feta cheese, and salt and pepper to taste, if desired. Drizzle on the dressing and toss gently.

FODMAP tip: *Five cherry tomatoes are equal to one low-FODMAP serving.*

Per serving: Calories: 346; Total fat: 18g; Total carbs: 39g; Fiber: 6g; Sugar: 7g; Protein: 10g; Sodium: 535mg

Vegetable Bolognese

Prep time: 5 minutes / Cook time: 28 minutes / Serves: 8

NUT-FREE, VEGETARIAN, QUICK-PREP

This vegetarian Bolognese is very hearty and filling. Serve it atop cooked spaghetti squash, gluten-free pasta, or polenta.

3 tablespoons olive oil

6 cups cubed eggplant (from about 1½ large eggplants)

1 medium red bell pepper, diced

1 medium zucchini, sliced, then cut into quarters

1 tablespoon tomato paste

1 (14.5-ounce) can diced tomatoes, no salt added, with juices

2 cups low-FODMAP pasta sauce

¼ cup dry red wine

½ cup canned coconut milk

¼ teaspoon ground nutmeg

1 tablespoon dried oregano

⅛ teaspoon kosher salt

¼ teaspoon freshly ground black pepper

½ cup shaved Parmesan cheese (optional)

1. In a large stockpot, heat the oil over medium heat. Add the eggplant and stir occasionally; cook for 2 minutes. Add the bell pepper and zucchini and cover; stir occasionally, cooking for 5 minutes.

2. Stir in the tomato paste until well combined. Cook for 1 minute. Add the canned tomatoes, pasta sauce, red wine, coconut milk, nutmeg, oregano, salt, and pepper. Bring to a boil. Reduce the heat. Cover and simmer for at least 20 minutes.

3. Add half the Parmesan cheese (if using) and stir. Serve in bowls and top each with remaining Parmesan cheese (if using).

Ingredient tip: See page 145 for a list of pasta sauces that are certified low-FODMAP or that are made with low-FODMAP ingredients.

Per serving: Calories: 148; Total fat: 9g; Total carbs: 15g; Fiber: 6g; Sugar: 8g; Protein: 2g; Sodium: 307mg

Lentil Burgers

Prep time: 2 minutes / **Cook time:** 10 minutes / **Serves:** 9

VEGAN OPTION, QUICK-PREP, UNDER 20 MINUTES

Canned lentils have a lower FODMAP content as long as you remember to drain and rinse them before using. A ½-cup, low-FODMAP serving of cooked lentils provides about 12 grams of protein and 9 grams of fiber, which makes these lentil burgers very hearty and nourishing.

1 teaspoon olive oil, plus more for cooking

8 ounces baby spinach

Juice of ½ lemon

½ teaspoon ground cumin

½ teaspoon kosher salt, divided

½ freshly ground black pepper

1 medium carrot, peeled and roughly chopped

½ cup walnuts

¼ cup sunflower seeds

2½ cups canned lentils, drained and rinsed

1 cup gluten-free plain bread crumbs

2 Flax Eggs (page 143)

2 tablespoons tomato paste

2 tablespoons Worcestershire sauce (or gluten-free tamari if vegan)

½ cup gluten-free low-FODMAP all-purpose flour

1. Heat the oil in a large nonstick skillet over medium heat. Add the spinach, lemon juice, cumin, ¼ teaspoon of salt, and pepper; stir until the spinach is wilted, about 3 minutes.

2. Using a food processor, finely chop the carrot, walnuts, and sunflower seeds, then transfer to a large bowl.

3. Add half the lentils to the food processor and pulse until mashed but not smooth. Transfer them to the large bowl along with the remaining lentils, then add the bread crumbs and the remaining ¼ teaspoon of salt.

4. In a small bowl, combine the flax eggs with the tomato paste and Worcestershire sauce. Pour the egg mixture into the bowl with the lentils and mix everything together with your hands. Sprinkle in the flour a little at a time as you continue to combine the ingredients. If the mixture seems too wet, add more flour as needed.

5. Form 9 individual flat patties.

6. In a skillet, heat a drizzle of oil over medium heat. Once the oil is heated, cook the burgers for 5 to 6 minutes on each side.

7. Serve on warm low-FODMAP buns with desired low-FODMAP toppings.

Continued ▶

Lentil Burgers
continued

FODMAP tip: *For those looking for vegan versions of Worcestershire sauce, try brands like Annie's Homegrown or Wizard's. Both the vegan versions as well as non-vegan versions like Lea & Perrins contain high-FODMAPs; however, Worcestershire sauce is currently rated low-FODMAP by the Monash University FODMAP Diet App at a serving of up to 2 tablespoons. That means the FODMAPs within that serving are at a low enough level to not cause issues. It's very rare that someone would consume 2 tablespoons of Worcestershire sauce in a sitting. Five tablespoons or more becomes high in the FODMAPs GOS and mannitol.*

Preparation tip: Some great low-FODMAP toppings for these burgers include baby arugula, fresh basil, roasted red bell peppers, soy cheese, cheddar cheese, shredded carrots, mustard, mayonnaise, or low-FODMAP barbeque sauce.

Per serving: Calories: 194; Total fat: 7g; Total carbs: 26g; Fiber: 8g; Sugar: 3g; Protein: 9g; Sodium: 237mg

Vietnamese Tempeh Bowl

Prep time: 5 minutes / **Cook time:** 10 minutes, plus 20 minutes to marinate the tempeh / **Serves:** 4

Tempeh is best when it's been dressed in a really good marinade, but it's hard to find any Asian-style marinades that aren't high-FODMAP. The marinade for this recipe has a Vietnamese flair that's perfect for tempeh.

2 tablespoons granulated sugar

½ cup seasoned rice vinegar

1 tablespoon fish sauce

1-inch piece fresh ginger, cut into 2 thick slices

1 tablespoon sesame oil

8 ounces tempeh

7 ounces rice noodles

1 tablespoon vegetable oil, for frying

1 large carrot, peeled and grated

2 cups fresh bean sprouts

1 jalapeño pepper, cored and thinly sliced

2 scallions, green parts only, chopped

3 tablespoons chopped fresh cilantro leaves

3 tablespoons chopped fresh mint leaves

¼ cup roasted peanuts, chopped

1 lime, quartered, for garnish

1. To make the marinade, in a large microwave-safe bowl, combine the sugar, rice vinegar, fish sauce, ginger, and sesame oil. Microwave in 30-second bursts, stirring each time, until the sugar has dissolved.

2. Cut the tempeh into thin slices, then add it to the bowl with the marinade. Allow to marinate for at least 20 minutes. Flip the pieces halfway through marinating.

3. Meanwhile, cook the rice noodles according to the package directions and set aside.

4. Heat the oil in a large skillet over medium heat. Once hot, fry the tempeh for about 2 minutes on each side. Remove the pan from the heat to prevent the residual marinade from burning. Using a wire mesh strainer, strain the leftover marinade still in the bowl to remove the ginger pieces; set aside.

5. Divide the rice noodles among 4 bowls. Top with the prepared tempeh, carrot, bean sprouts, jalapeño pepper, scallions, cilantro, mint, peanuts, and lime wedges. After squeezing the fresh limes, pour any leftover marinade into the bowls, if desired.

Make-ahead tip: Make the marinade ahead of time and toss it with the tempeh and cover in the refrigerator for 2 to 24 hours. If the tempeh isn't fully immersed in the marinade, flip the pieces halfway through.

Per serving: Calories: 434; Total fat: 14g; Total carbs: 63g; Fiber: 3g; Sugar: 10g; Protein: 18g; Sodium: 585mg

Pad Thai Bowl with Peanut Sauce and Crispy Tofu

Prep time: 15 minutes / Cook time: 15 minutes / Serves: 6

VEGETARIAN

Instead of a typical stir-fried pad thai, this recipe calls for the noodles to be cold (though you can certainly keep the noodles warm if you'd like). Pad thai typically contains high-FODMAP ingredients, but you can avoid them and still have plenty of flavor to go around.

14 ounces extra-firm tofu, drained, pressed, and cut into cubes

8 ounces pad thai-style rice noodles

1-inch piece fresh ginger, cut into 2 thick slices

¼ cup peanut butter

Juice from ½ medium navel orange

Juice from 1 large lime (about 3 tablespoons)

2 tablespoons soy sauce

1½ tablespoons honey

3 tablespoons toasted sesame oil

½ teaspoon cayenne pepper

½ teaspoon kosher salt

5 to 6 tablespoons cornstarch

1 tablespoon vegetable oil, for frying

1 red bell pepper, thinly sliced

1 cup shredded red cabbage

1 cup shredded carrots

3 scallions, green parts only, sliced

½ cup fresh basil, chopped

1 tablespoon finely chopped fresh jalapeño pepper

½ cup roasted, crushed peanuts (optional)

6 lime wedges

1. Cook the noodles according to the directions on the package. Drain, run under cold water, cover, and put in the refrigerator.

2. While the noodles are cooking, make the peanut sauce by combining the ginger, peanut butter, orange juice, lime juice, soy sauce, honey, sesame oil, cayenne pepper, and salt in a blender or food processor and blend.

3. Put the cubed tofu in a zip-top bag. Add the cornstarch 1 tablespoon at a time, closing the bag each time to shake it and coat the tofu.

4. Heat the oil in a large skillet over medium heat. Add the tofu and fry until golden and crispy, 2 to 3 minutes per side.

5. Put the bell pepper, cabbage, carrots, scallions, basil, and jalapeño pepper into a large serving bowl. Toss to combine. Add the chilled noodles and tofu to the serving bowl and toss again. Pour the peanut sauce over the top and toss gently to combine. Divide among bowls and garnish with the roasted peanuts and a lime wedge.

Preparation tip: To drain the tofu, line a plate with paper towels and put the tofu block on top of the paper towels. Then put another layer of paper towels on top of the tofu. Put a heavy cutting board or heavy pot on top of the paper towels and use heavy books or cans to weigh it down further. Let it drain for 30 minutes to 1 hour, then remove the weight and drain off the excess liquid. Pat the tofu dry with more paper towels.

Per serving: Calories: 399; Total fat: 18g; Total carbs: 52g; Fiber: 3g; Sugar: 10g; Protein: 11g; Sodium: 638mg

Hawaiian Tofu Tacos

Prep time: 7 minutes / Cook time: 20 minutes / Serves: 4

NUT-FREE, VEGETARIAN, QUICK-PREP, UNDER 30 MINUTES

Most Hawaiian tacos offered in restaurants come with high-FODMAP ingredients. You can avoid the meat and the FODMAPs with this delicious vegetarian recipe, complete with crispy tofu, sweet pineapple, crunchy cabbage, and a homemade barbecue sauce recipe that will make your mouth water!

1 (14-ounce) block firm tofu

5 to 6 tablespoons cornstarch

1 cup Fody Foods™ Low-FODMAP Ketchup

¼ cup apple cider vinegar

2 tablespoons packed brown sugar

1 tablespoon honey

½ tablespoon Worcestershire sauce (see FODMAP Tip on page 68)

½ tablespoon freshly squeezed lemon juice

1 tablespoon vegetable oil

2 cups fresh pineapple chunks

2 cups shredded red cabbage

¼ cup chopped fresh cilantro, for garnish

1. Drain the tofu (see the Preparation tip on page 71).

2. Cut the tofu into ½-inch cubes and put it in a medium bowl. Add the cornstarch, 1 tablespoon at a time; toss to coat each cube of tofu. Set aside.

3. For the barbecue sauce, whisk together the ketchup, apple cider vinegar, brown sugar, honey, Worcestershire sauce, and lemon juice in a medium saucepan over medium heat. Once it is bubbling rapidly, reduce the heat to low and simmer until thickened, about 10 minutes.

4. Add the oil to a nonstick skillet over medium-high heat; add the tofu. Fry for 2 to 3 minutes on each side until crispy. Set the tofu aside on a plate.

5. Wipe the skillet clean of oil or tofu pieces. Return the skillet to medium heat and add half of the barbecue sauce. Add the tofu, then cover with the remaining sauce. Cook for another 1 to 2 minutes, then remove from the heat.

6. Divide the tofu, pineapple, and red cabbage among 4 low-FODMAP tortillas. Garnish with the cilantro.

FODMAP tip: Be sure to divide the cabbage evenly for this recipe. Three-quarters of a cup is equal to one low-FODMAP serving.

Per serving: Calories: 381; Total fat: 13g; Total carbs: 52g; Fiber: 5g; Sugar: 34g; Protein: 17g; Sodium: 618mg

Moroccan Eggplant Tagine

Prep time: 5 minutes / **Cook time:** 30 minutes, plus 10 minutes to release the pressure / **Serves:** 4

VEGETARIAN, QUICK-PREP

A tagine is a clay or ceramic cooking vessel, but an Instant Pot or pressure cooker can work just as well. This low-FODMAP recipe will fill your home with an intoxicating smell of spices that will make you swoon!

1 red bell pepper, chopped

½ tablespoon Garlic-Infused Oil (page 134)

1-inch piece fresh ginger, peeled and minced

2 teaspoons ground cumin

2 teaspoons ground turmeric

2 teaspoons ground coriander

½ teaspoon ground cinnamon

¼ teaspoon saffron threads

1 (14.5-ounce) can crushed tomatoes

4 cups low-FODMAP vegetable broth

1 cup canned chickpeas, drained and rinsed

1 teaspoon honey

¼ cup raisins

⅓ cup unsalted macadamia nuts

¼ teaspoon kosher salt

½ teaspoon freshly ground black pepper

4 cups chopped eggplant

2 medium sweet potatoes, peeled and cut into bite-size pieces

½ preserved lemon or 2 tablespoons lemon zest

½ teaspoon dried mint (optional)

1. In a large skillet, sauté the bell pepper in the oil for 2 minutes. Add the ginger, cumin, turmeric, coriander, cinnamon, and saffron and cook for another minute. Stir, then add the crushed tomatoes, broth, chickpeas, honey, raisins, macadamia nuts, salt, and pepper. Stir in the chopped eggplant, sweet potatoes, and preserved lemon.

2. Cover, set the vent on your Instant Pot to sealing, and cook for 20 minutes at high pressure. Allow 10 minutes for natural pressure release, then manually release the remaining steam. For a pressure cooker, close the lid, cook on high pressure for 16 minutes, then let the pressure release naturally for 10 minutes. Release the remaining pressure manually.

3. Add the dried mint (if using) and adjust the seasonings if necessary.

Serving tip: Serve with up to 6 ounces of strained Greek yogurt or 1 tablespoon of lactose-free sour cream. This dish also tastes delicious served atop quinoa or rice with crumbled feta.

Per serving: Calories: 267; Total fat: 5g; Total carbs: 51g; Fiber: 12g; Sugar: 21g; Protein: 7g; Sodium: 440mg

Creamy Polenta with Mushrooms

Prep time: 2 minutes / Cook time: 10 minutes / Serves: 5

NUT-FREE, VEGAN, QUICK-PREP, UNDER 30 MINUTES

This dish is creamy, savory, and comforting on a cold day. I love the smoothness of the polenta with the tender mushrooms and creamy coconut. Enjoy a hearty serving for a meal or have a smaller serving as a side dish.

1 (6.5-ounce) can mushroom caps and stems, drained and rinsed

½ teaspoon dried sage

1 tablespoon olive oil

⅛ teaspoon kosher salt

¼ teaspoon freshly ground black pepper

1 (18-ounce) tube polenta

¼ cup canned lite coconut milk

½ cup low-FODMAP vegetable broth, warmed

1. In a medium saucepan over medium heat, combine the mushrooms, sage, oil, salt, and pepper and cook for 2 minutes, stirring occasionally. Add the polenta, coconut milk, and broth, and stir to combine.

2. Use a fork to mash down the polenta and stir again. Cook for 4 to 6 minutes or until heated through. (For a creamier consistency, add another ¼ cup of coconut milk.)

3. Divide among 5 bowls and serve immediately.

Preparation tip: If you don't have dried sage, dried oregano and dried thyme are just as lovely.

Per serving: Calories: 182; Total fat: 4g; Total carbs: 32g; Fiber: 3g; Sugar: 3g; Protein: 5g; Sodium: 627mg

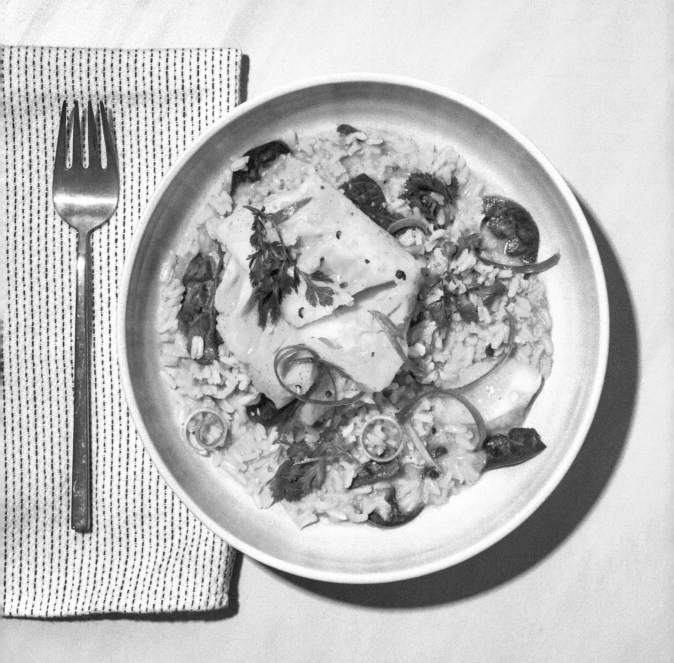

Halibut in Coconut Curry Sauce, page 83

CHAPTER 5

Fish and Seafood

Asian-Style Fusion Salmon

Prep time: 5 minutes / Cook time: 20 minutes / Serves: 4

DAIRY-FREE, NUT-FREE, QUICK-PREP, UNDER 30 MINUTES

This recipe was inspired by the time I went to Melbourne, Australia. Asian fusion is a popular cuisine in Melbourne, and I was impressed by the variety of Asian-style fare, flavors, and textures. Salmon is already a flavorful fish and is so delectable paired with this sauce.

2 pounds salmon fillets

1 tablespoon rice vinegar

1 tablespoon sesame oil

2 tablespoons soy sauce

¼ cup maple syrup

1 tablespoon freshly grated ginger

1 teaspoon sriracha

1 tablespoon thinly sliced scallions, green parts only

1. Preheat the oven to 375°F.

2. Put the salmon in an aluminum foil–lined baking dish, using enough foil to cover the salmon.

3. In a small bowl, mix together the rice vinegar, sesame oil, soy sauce, maple syrup, ginger, sriracha, and scallions. Mix well to combine.

4. Slowly pour the sauce over the salmon. Pull the foil over the salmon and crumple the seams securely together. Be sure to cover the salmon completely.

5. Bake for 16 to 20 minutes. When the salmon is done, it should flake easily with a fork, or reach an internal temperature of 145°F.

Make-ahead tip: For a more infused flavor, put the salmon in an airtight container or zip-top bag and pour in the marinade and cover; refrigerate for 30 minutes.

Per serving: Calories: 448; Total fat: 21g; Total carbs: 15g; Fiber: 0g; Sugar: 12g; Protein: 43g; Sodium: 473mg

Greek-Style Shrimp Pasta

Prep time: 5 minutes / **Cook time:** 20 minutes / **Serves:** 4

NUT-FREE, QUICK-PREP, UNDER 30 MINUTES

Kale, shrimp, and feta are the shining stars of this delicious take on Greek food. It may become one of your new go-to dishes!

1 pound gluten-free and low-FODMAP fettuccine

4 Roma tomatoes, diced

¼ teaspoon kosher salt, divided

¼ teaspoon dried oregano

¼ teaspoon red pepper flakes

½ tablespoon Garlic-Infused Oil (page 134)

1 medium bunch curly kale, stemmed, sliced thinly (about 5 cups)

1 pound large shrimp, peeled, deveined

1 tablespoon freshly squeezed lemon juice

1 tablespoon butter

2½ ounces crumbled feta (about ½ cup)

1. Cook the pasta according to the package directions.

2. While the pasta is boiling, heat a medium nonstick pan over medium heat. Add the tomatoes and ⅛ teaspoon of salt. Cook for 5 minutes, stirring frequently.

3. After the pasta has boiled, carefully pour ½ cup of pasta water into a glass measuring cup. Set aside. Drain the pasta and put it in a serving bowl. Set aside.

4. Add the oregano, red pepper flakes, and oil to the pan with the tomatoes, and stir for 1 minute. Next, add the kale, 1 cup at a time, stirring frequently.

5. Add ¼ cup of the reserved pasta water, stirring occasionally for about 2 minutes. Add the remaining pasta water and stir for another 2 minutes.

6. Add the shrimp, lemon juice, butter, and remaining ⅛ teaspoon of salt and continue to stir. Cook for 3 to 5 minutes.

7. Add the contents of the pan to the bowl of pasta. Add the feta and toss gently once or twice. Serve immediately.

Preparation tip: Buy shrimp that have been peeled and deveined to save time.

Per serving: Calories: 459; Total fat: 21g; Total carbs: 40g; Fiber: 6g; Sugar: 5g; Protein: 34g; Sodium: 587mg

Scallops with Brown Butter Sage Sauce, Pine Nuts, and Butternut Squash

Prep time: 5 minutes / Cook time: 15 minutes / Serves: 4

QUICK-PREP, UNDER 30 MINUTES

Sage is probably my favorite herb, and I especially love it with butternut squash. This recipe is great as a side dish or makes a lovely meal with low-FODMAP pasta.

3 tablespoons unsalted butter, cut into small pieces

3 sprigs fresh sage

1⅓ cups diced (bite-size pieces) butternut squash

2 tablespoons pine nuts

1 pound sea scallops (dry scallops are best)

¼ teaspoon kosher salt

⅛ teaspoon freshly ground black pepper

Nonstick cooking spray

4 cups cooked low-FODMAP and gluten-free pasta

1. Heat a 14-inch skillet over medium heat. Put the butter in the skillet and whisk frequently for 2 minutes. Remove from the heat. Add the sage, and whisk continuously for 2 minutes. Add the butternut squash to the pan and return to the burner, heating to medium-high.

2. Use a spoon to coat all the pieces of squash with the butter and spread the pieces around the pan in an even layer. Cook for 4 minutes, then add the pine nuts, flip the squash, and cook for another 6 minutes, until tender. Then push the butternut squash and pine nuts to one side of the pan.

3. While the squash is cooking, season the scallops with the salt and pepper. Spray the other side of the pan lightly with nonstick cooking spray and add the scallops. Cook for 3 minutes, then flip the scallops, cover, and cook for an additional 3 minutes. Remove everything from the pan and serve with the pasta.

Ingredient tip: Make sure that the gluten-free pasta is low-FODMAP (i.e., no legume flour [besan, soy, or urid]).

Per serving: Calories: 426; Total fat: 13g; Total carbs: 53g; Fiber: 2g; Sugar: 1g; Protein: 24g; Sodium: 196mg

Sushi Roll Bowl

Prep time: 20 minutes / Cook time: 20 minutes / Serves: 4

DAIRY-FREE, NUT-FREE

I love sushi, but if raw fish isn't your thing, try crabmeat, cooked shrimp, or scallops for this super-delish recipe. Be sure to purchase real crabmeat to avoid the Polyol sorbitol. When purchasing pickled ginger, please read the label to ensure it does not contain high-fructose corn syrup.

2 cups sushi rice

2 cups cold water

5 tablespoons rice wine vinegar, divided

1 tablespoon sugar

½ teaspoon fine sea salt

1 cup diced cucumber

1 medium carrot, peeled and sliced thin

1 radish, sliced thin

1 sheet nori, cut into ⅛-inch strips, divided (optional)

16 ounces lump crabmeat (or cooked shrimp or scallops), divided

½ medium avocado, cut into eighths

3 tablespoons low-sodium soy sauce (or tamari if gluten-free)

2 tablespoons chopped pickled ginger

2 tablespoons toasted sesame seeds

1 cup frozen edamame, shelled, thawed, and divided (optional)

2 tablespoons seaweed (nori) flakes (optional)

1 scallion, green parts only, chopped (optional)

1. Rinse the rice in a large mesh colander until the water runs clear. Put the rice in a medium saucepot and cover with the cold water. Bring to a boil. Reduce the heat to low, cover, and simmer for 15 minutes. Remove from the heat and let stand, covered, for 15 minutes.

2. While the rice cooks, in a small microwave-safe bowl, combine 3 tablespoons of rice wine vinegar with the sugar and salt; stir until dissolved. Microwave for 1 minute. Combine the vinegar mixture and rice in a large bowl and toss to mix. Let cool for 5 minutes.

3. Divide the rice evenly between 4 serving bowls and top each with the cucumber, carrot, radish, nori strips (if using), and crabmeat, then 2 slices of avocado.

4. In a small bowl, whisk together the remaining 2 tablespoons of rice vinegar and soy sauce. Drizzle over the top of each bowl and garnish with the pickled ginger and sesame seeds. If desired, top each bowl with ¼ cup edamame, ½ tablespoon of seaweed flakes, and scallions.

FODMAP tip: *An eighth of a whole medium avocado is a low-FODMAP serving. Use a digital scale to measure out 30 grams per serving.*

Per serving: Calories: 605; Total fat: 8g; Total carbs: 101g; Fiber: 3g; Sugar: 5g; Protein: 31g; Sodium: 1225mg

Spicy Salmon

Prep time: 5 minutes / Cook time: 10 minutes / Serves: 2

DAIRY-FREE, NUT-FREE, QUICK-PREP, UNDER 30 MINUTES

This salmon recipe is full of flavor and goes well with my Quinoa Spinach (page 40) or Colorful Crunchy Salad (page 50).

For the rub

- **1 teaspoon asafetida powder**
- **1 teaspoon sea salt**
- **½ teaspoon ground paprika**
- **½ teaspoon dried dill**
- **½ teaspoon dried thyme**
- **½ teaspoon ground ginger**
- **⅛ teaspoon cayenne pepper**
- **⅛ teaspoon freshly ground black pepper**

For the salmon

- **2 (3-ounce) salmon fillets**
- **1 tablespoon extra-virgin olive oil**

1. In a small bowl, combine the asafetida powder, salt, paprika, dill, thyme, ginger, cayenne pepper, and black pepper. Store in an airtight container in the cupboard or freezer.

2. Brush the salmon with the oil. Sprinkle with two-thirds of the seasoning and rub it in (reserve the remaining rub for another time). Cook the fish over a hot grill or broil it about 6 inches away from the broiler for 6 to 10 minutes, until it flakes easily with a fork. Serve immediately.

Ingredient tip: If you'd like to use another fish, try red snapper, flounder, tilapia, shrimp, or scallops.

Per serving: Calories: 248; Total fat: 20g; Total carbs: 2g; Fiber: 1g; Sugar: 0g; Protein: 16g; Sodium: 311mg

Halibut in Coconut Curry Sauce

Prep time: 5 minutes / Cook time: 20 minutes / Serves: 4

DAIRY-FREE, NUT-FREE, QUICK-PREP, UNDER 30 MINUTES

This healthy and fragrant meal comes together very easily and quickly. You'll love how delicate the fish becomes from sitting in the sauce and the smell of the coconut and lemongrass.

2 teaspoons vegetable oil

2 teaspoons curry powder

1 tablespoon lemongrass paste

2 cups low-FODMAP broth

½ cup light unsweetened canned coconut milk

¾ teaspoon sea salt, divided, plus more for seasoning

4 cups baby spinach

4 (6-ounce) halibut fillets, skin removed

½ cup coarsely chopped fresh cilantro leaves

2 scallions, green parts only, thinly sliced

2 tablespoons freshly squeezed lime juice

Freshly ground black pepper

2 cups cooked brown rice

1. In a large sauté pan, heat the oil over moderate heat. Add the curry powder, and stir in the lemongrass paste and cook for 1 minute. Add the broth, coconut milk, and ½ teaspoon of salt, and reduce the heat to low. Simmer for 5 minutes.

2. While the sauce is simmering, put the spinach in a microwave-safe bowl covered loosely with a lid or a piece of plastic wrap. Microwave on high until all the leaves have turned dark green and are wilted, 2 to 3 minutes. Set aside.

3. Place the halibut fillets on a plate and season both sides with the remaining ¼ teaspoon of salt. Arrange the fish in the pan and ladle the sauce over the fish to coat. Cover and cook until the fish flakes easily with a fork, about 7 minutes.

4. Stir the cilantro, scallions, and lime juice into the sauce and season with salt and pepper to taste. Cook for 2 minutes.

5. Reheat the cooked rice in the microwave, 1 to 2 minutes.

6. Arrange the rice and then a pile of steamed spinach in the bottom of 4 bowls. Top with the fish fillets. Ladle the sauce over the fish and serve.

Ingredient tip: When buying spices like curry, make sure it does not contain added high-FODMAPs such as onion or garlic or "spices," which could also be onion or garlic.

Per serving: Calories: 418; Total fat: 10g; Total carbs: 27g; Fiber: 2g; Sugar: 1g; Protein: 50g; Sodium: 320mg

Cod Puttanesca

Prep time: 10 minutes / Cook time: 20 minutes / Serves: 4

DAIRY-FREE, NUT-FREE

Puttanesca is an Italian-style pasta dish that was invented in Naples in the mid-20th century. The ingredients typically include tomatoes, olive oil, anchovies, olives, capers, and garlic. This low-FODMAP version served over fish doesn't need high-FODMAP garlic to make it taste so good!

1 cup gluten-free all-purpose low-FODMAP flour, for dusting

1½ pounds cod, cut into chunks

Sea salt

Freshly ground black pepper

¼ cup olive or vegetable oil

1 (14.5-ounce) can salt-free diced tomatoes

12 green pitted olives, sliced

12 black pitted olives, sliced

2 tablespoons capers

¼ cup white cooking wine

¼ teaspoon red pepper flakes

¼ cup chopped fresh parsley

1. Gather 2 shallow bowls. Leave one bowl empty and pour the flour into the other bowl. Put each piece of fish in the first bowl and season lightly with salt and pepper, then place them in the second bowl and dredge with the flour. Repeat until finished with all of the fish.

2. Heat the oil in a large sauté pan or skillet over medium-high heat. When hot, add the fish and fry until golden, 2 to 4 minutes per side. Set aside on a serving plate.

3. Add the tomatoes, olives, capers, wine, red pepper flakes, and parsley to the pan, and cook for 5 to 7 minutes, stirring occasionally. Serve over the fish with polenta, gluten-free pasta, or rice.

Ingredient tip: When buying canned tomatoes be sure that no onion, garlic, "spices" or "natural flavorings" are present among the ingredients.

Per serving: Calories: 414; Total fat: 18g; Total carbs: 25g; Fiber: 4g; Sugar: 0g; Protein: 33g; Sodium: 482mg

Shrimp with Polenta

Prep time: 2 minutes / Cook time: 20 minutes / Serves: 4

NUT-FREE, QUICK-PREP, UNDER 30 MINUTES

This dish is super delicious in so many ways! From the smooth polenta, to the herbs and red pepper flakes, to the succulent shrimp cooked in wine and tomatoes.

1 (18-ounce) tube polenta

¼ cup low-FODMAP milk

2 tablespoons olive oil

¼ pound pancetta, chopped (optional)

¼ teaspoon dried sage

¼ teaspoon dried thyme

¼ teaspoon dried basil

¼ teaspoon dried oregano

⅛ teaspoon red pepper flakes

1 (14.5-ounce) can diced tomatoes in juice

¼ cup white cooking wine

1 pound large shrimp, peeled and deveined

4 ounces shaved Parmesan cheese, divided

¼ teaspoon freshly ground black pepper

3 tablespoons chopped fresh parsley, divided

1. Cook the polenta according to the package instructions in a heavy medium saucepan with the low-FODMAP milk. Stir frequently and cook until thickened and creamy, about 5 minutes. Remove from the heat.

2. Pour the oil into a 10-inch heavy skillet over medium heat. Cook the pancetta (if using), sage, thyme, basil, oregano, and red pepper flakes, stirring frequently, 2 to 3 minutes. Add the tomatoes with their juice and wine; simmer for 5 minutes. Add the shrimp and cook, flipping over halfway, until the shrimp are just cooked through, about 3 minutes.

3. Spoon the polenta into shallow bowls and top with the Parmesan cheese, then add the shrimp mixture. Season with the pepper and top with the parsley.

Preparation tip: Try cooking the polenta with low-FODMAP chicken broth instead of low-FODMAP milk.

Per serving: Calories: 547; Total fat: 15g; Total carbs: 44g; Fiber: 3g; Sugar: 4g; Protein: 38g; Sodium: 1097mg

Cajun Fish Stew

Prep time: 10 minutes / Cook time: 15 minutes / Serves: 4

DAIRY-FREE, NUT-FREE, ONE POT, UNDER 30 MINUTES

Looking for something to make on a cold day? Try this super healthy and spicy stew to warm you up. It's very filling and one of my favorite go-to recipes because it's so easy and flavorful. It tastes especially great when served over rice prepared with a little bit of butter.

1 tablespoon olive oil

⅔ cup chopped fresh parsley

½ teaspoon cayenne pepper

½ teaspoon sweet paprika

¼ teaspoon dried oregano

¼ teaspoon dried thyme

¼ teaspoon freshly ground black pepper

1 (14.5-ounce) can salt-free, whole or diced tomatoes with their juices

2 teaspoons tomato paste

8 ounces clam juice

½ cup dry white wine

½ pound shrimp

1½ pounds tilapia fillets, cut into 2-inch pieces

Sea salt

1 lemon, cut into wedges (optional)

1. Heat the oil in a large, thick-bottomed pot over medium-high heat. Add the parsley, cayenne pepper, paprika, oregano, thyme, and pepper and stir for 1 minute. Add the tomatoes and tomato paste, and cook for 10 minutes, stirring every 2 minutes.

2. Add the clam juice, wine, shrimp, and fish. Cover and bring to a simmer for about 5 minutes, until the shrimp is opaque and the fish is cooked through and easily flakes apart. Add salt to taste. Serve with the lemon wedges (if using).

Substitution tip: Tilapia works best for this recipe, but you can also try cod, halibut, or red snapper.

Ingredient tip: If you cannot find clam juice, you can use shrimp or shellfish stock as long as it does not contain high-FODMAPs.

Per serving: Calories: 307; Total fat: 6g; Total carbs: 9g; Fiber: 1g; Sugar: 3g; Protein: 44g; Sodium: 331mg

Easy Weeknight Fish Tacos

Prep time: 10 minutes / **Cook time:** 15 minutes / **Serves:** 4

NUT-FREE, UNDER 30 MINUTES

Fish tacos are an all-around favorite and so easy to make. For a perfect, fresh, and delicious match, try my dreamy Creamy Cilantro Taco Sauce with these tasty fish tacos.

1 tablespoon chili powder

½ teaspoon ground cumin

1 teaspoon dried oregano

1 teaspoon ground paprika

½ teaspoon sea salt

½ teaspoon freshly ground black pepper

1½ pounds tilapia fillets

1 tablespoon olive oil

8 (6-inch) corn tortillas

1 small tomato, chopped (optional)

2 cups iceberg lettuce, shredded (optional)

Creamy Cilantro Taco Sauce (page 131; optional)

1 small lime, cut in wedges, for serving

1. Preheat the oven to 400°F. Line a pan with parchment paper.

2. Combine the chili powder, cumin, oregano, paprika, salt, and pepper in a small bowl and set aside.

3. Brush the fish fillets with the oil. Rub the spices and herb mix onto the fish fillets. Place the fish on the prepared pan. Bake for 12 to 15 minutes or until flaky and cooked through.

4. Heat the tortillas in a medium pan over low heat.

5. Cut the fish into 8 chunks and divide them between the tortillas. If desired, top with the tomato, lettuce, and creamy cilantro taco sauce, and serve with a lime wedge.

FODMAP tip: *When buying spices such as chili powder, make sure it doesn't contain garlic or other "spices," which could also be garlic or onion.*

Per serving: Calories: 285; Total fat: 7g; Total carbs: 23g; Fiber: 4g; Sugar: 1g; Protein: 35g; Sodium: 336mg

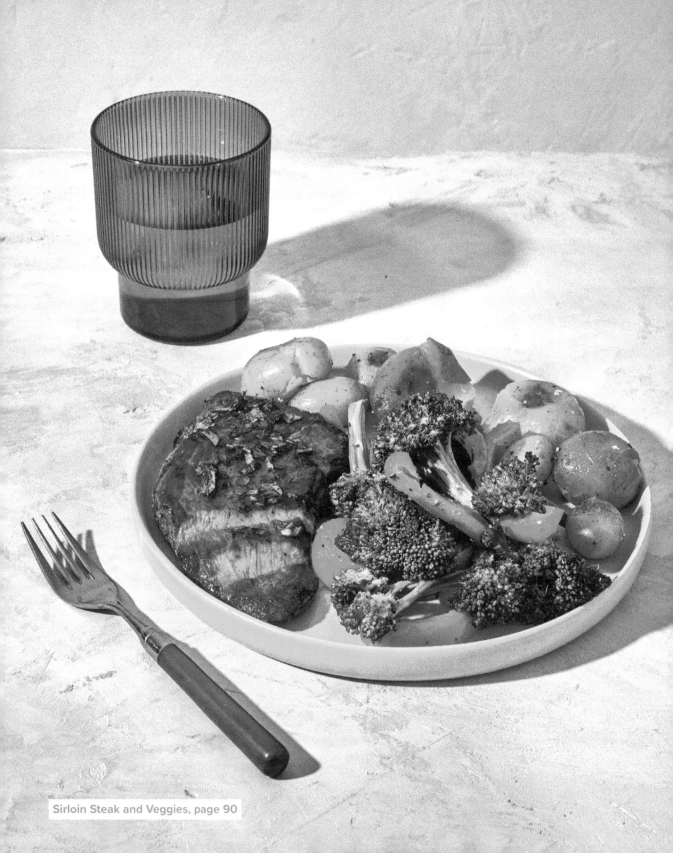

Sirloin Steak and Veggies, page 90

CHAPTER 6

Poultry and Meat

Sirloin Steak and Veggies

Prep time: 5 minutes / **Cook time:** 25 minutes / **Serves:** 5

ONE POT, NUT-FREE

This one's for the meat and potato lovers! There's nothing better than tender potatoes, juicy steak, and flavorful red peppers. Go ahead, enjoy with one low-FODMAP serving (one glass, or about 5 ounces) of red wine!

2½ cups broccoli florets

1 medium red bell pepper, cored and cut into ½-inch slices

2 tablespoons olive oil

½ teaspoon dried thyme

½ teaspoon dried oregano

¾ teaspoon kosher salt, divided

¾ teaspoon freshly ground black pepper, divided

2 pounds small potatoes (such as red potatoes)

2 pounds (1-inch-thick) top sirloin steak, patted dry

1. Preheat the oven to 425°F. Line a large baking tray with parchment paper.

2. Put the broccoli and bell pepper in a medium bowl. Add the oil, thyme, oregano, ¼ teaspoon of salt, and ¼ teaspoon of black pepper. Toss to combine.

3. Place the broccoli florets and bell pepper on the baking tray and roast for 17 minutes. Once done, remove from the oven and set aside on a dish or in a serving bowl.

4. While the vegetables are roasting, fill a large pot with water and add the potatoes. Boil for 12 to 15 minutes, until they have a cooked outer edge and a raw middle. Immediately put the potatoes into a bowl of cold water.

5. Season both sides of the steaks with ¼ teaspoon of salt and ¼ teaspoon of pepper. Preheat the oven to broil. Put the steak and potatoes on the baking sheet. Season the potatoes with the remaining ¼ teaspoon of salt and ¼ teaspoon of pepper. Put into the oven for 4 to 6 minutes per side for medium-rare, or until it reaches your desired doneness.

6. Divide the steak, broccoli, red peppers, and potatoes among 5 plates. Serve immediately.

FODMAP tip: A ¾-cup serving of broccoli florets is equal to 1 low-FODMAP serving.

Per serving: Calories: 438; Total fat: 13g; Total carbs: 33g; Fiber: 6g; Sugar: 4g; Protein: 46g; Sodium: 374mg

Turkey and Pork Meatballs

Prep time: 10 minutes / **Cook time:** 30 minutes, plus 7 minutes to release the pressure / **Serves:** 4

ONE POT, NUT-FREE

Made in an Instant Pot, these meatballs are done quickly and have a moist texture. Make sure to use plain bread crumbs that contain no added high-FODMAP ingredients. Serve these delicious meatballs with low-FODMAP pasta and sauce, rice, quinoa, "zoodles" and sauce, or atop creamy polenta.

½ **pound lean ground turkey**

½ **pound ground pork**

¼ **cup sliced water chestnuts, diced**

2 **tablespoons finely chopped parsley**

1 **large egg**

½ **teaspoon Worcestershire sauce**

1 **tablespoon lactose-free milk (full-fat if possible)**

½ **cup gluten-free plain bread crumbs**

½ **cup grated Parmesan cheese**

½ **teaspoon kosher salt**

¼ **teaspoon freshly ground black pepper**

¼ **teaspoon red pepper flakes**

2 **tablespoons olive oil**

½ **cup low-FODMAP chicken broth**

1. In a large mixing bowl, combine the ground turkey, ground pork, water chestnuts, parsley, egg, Worcestershire sauce, milk, bread crumbs, Parmesan cheese, salt, pepper, and red pepper flakes. Mix well with your hands until all the ingredients are evenly combined.

2. Take about 2 tablespoons of meat and form a meatball. Repeat the process until you have 12 meatballs total.

3. Set the Instant Pot to Sauté on high heat and pour in the olive oil. Once the oil is hot, brown the meatballs for 1 to 2 minutes on each side, or until they become golden. Remove the meatballs from the pot.

4. Scrape any brown leftover bits from the bottom of the pot. Place a trivet in the bottom of the pot and then put the meatballs on top. Pour in the broth.

5. Cover with a lid and cook on Manual high pressure for 7 minutes. Turn the venting knob to the sealing position.

6. Naturally release the pressure for 5 to 7 minutes. Then switch the knob to the venting position and release the steam.

Preparation tip: If you don't have an Instant Pot, line a 13-by-9-inch pan with aluminum foil sprayed with nonstick cooking spray, then bake the meatballs in the oven at 400°F for 18 to 22 minutes.

Per serving: Calories: 343; Total fat: 24g; Total carbs: 6g; Fiber: 0g; Sugar: 1g; Protein: 28g; Sodium: 550mg

One Pot Creamy Mexican Mac 'n' Cheese

Prep time: 5 minutes / Cook time: 25 minutes / Serves: 6

ONE POT, NUT-FREE

This recipe is a family favorite at our house, and we never have any left-overs. Red kidney or pinto beans are usually used in Mexican dishes, but a low-FODMAP serving of chickpeas takes the show. Add the spices and creaminess of the cheese and your senses will be wowed!

1 teaspoon olive oil

1 pound ground lean beef or ground bison

1 red bell pepper, cored and diced

1 teaspoon chili powder

1½ teaspoons ground cumin

1 teaspoon dried oregano

4 cups low-FODMAP beef or chicken broth

Kosher salt

Freshly ground black pepper

¾ cup chickpeas, drained and rinsed

10 ounces gluten-free and low-FODMAP elbow macaroni

1 cup low-FODMAP pasta sauce

2 ounces lactose-free cream cheese

6 tablespoons shredded cheddar cheese

⅓ cup fresh cilantro, chopped

1. Heat the olive oil in a 14-inch pot over medium-high heat. Add the ground beef and bell pepper and cook for 5 to 6 minutes.

2. Add the chili powder, cumin, oregano, broth, salt, pepper, chickpeas, and macaroni to the pot. Stir to combine.

3. Bring to a simmer, then cover the pot and cook for 12 to 13 minutes or until the pasta is tender. Uncover the pot, add the pasta sauce, and cook for an additional 3 to 4 minutes.

4. Transfer the pasta mixture to a large serving bowl. Add the cream cheese and mix until the cream cheese has melted evenly throughout the pasta.

5. Top each bowl with 1 tablespoon of shredded cheese, and garnish with the cilantro.

Ingredient tip: I used Prego® Sensitive Recipe Traditional Italian Sauce for this recipe. For this sauce, a ½-cup serving per person has been tested to be low-FODMAP. If you use a different low-FODMAP brand, be sure to check the label for serving sizes.

Per serving: Calories: 431; Total fat: 15g; Total carbs: 48g; Fiber: 4g; Sugar: 4g; Protein: 26g; Sodium: 614mg

Chicken Vitality Bowl

Prep time: 2 minutes / Cook time: 25 minutes / Serves: 2

QUICK-PREP, UNDER 30 MINUTES, VEGETARIAN OPTION

Inspired by a bowl I had at a café in Solana Beach in San Diego, I've recreated this recipe to be low-FODMAP just for you. Dig in for the pesto, warm chicken, and Parmesan! Vegetarian? Try firm tofu instead of chicken.

1 pound skinless, boneless chicken breast

1 tablespoon olive oil

⅛ teaspoon kosher salt

1 cup rice, cooked

1 tablespoon Pesto Sauce (page 130) or low-FODMAP pesto, divided

3 cups spinach

2 tablespoons slivered almonds, toasted

½ tablespoon freshly squeezed lemon juice, or more

½ cup shaved Parmesan cheese, divided

1. Preheat the oven to 400°F.

2. Rub the chicken breast with the olive oil and sprinkle both sides with the salt. Put the chicken on a broiler pan and bake for 10 minutes. Flip the chicken and cook until no longer pink in the center and the juices run clear, about 15 minutes more.

3. Meanwhile, reheat the rice in a pan over low heat, stirring occasionally, 1 to 2 minutes.

4. Once the chicken is cooked and cooled, cut it into cubes and toss into a large bowl with the heated rice. Add the pesto sauce, spinach, almonds, lemon juice, and Parmesan cheese. Toss to combine and serve immediately.

Make-ahead tip: To save time, make your rice ahead on your meal prep night and refrigerate or freeze. Chicken can also be made ahead of time on your meal prep night. After cooking, transfer to a glass airtight container in the refrigerator and use within 3 to 4 days.

Per serving: Calories: 587; Total fat: 22g; Total carbs: 32g; Fiber: 2g; Sugar: 1g; Protein: 64g; Sodium: 667mg

Filet Mignon with a Blueberry Glaze

Prep time: 15 minutes / Cook time: 10 minutes / Serves: 2

NUT-FREE, UNDER 30 MINUTES

One night at a lovely Italian restaurant, I had a dish just like this one. It was the most exquisite pairing of flavors! It seems like a super fancy dish, but it's easy to make, and everyone loves it.

2 (6- to 8-ounce) tenderloin beef filets (roughly 2 inches thick)

½ teaspoon kosher salt, divided

½ teaspoon freshly ground black pepper, divided

½ cup fresh blueberries, mashed

½ cup dry red wine (such as Chianti, Cabernet Sauvignon, Pinot Noir, Shiraz/Syrah)

2 teaspoons honey

Juice and rind from half a lemon

1 tablespoon brown sugar, packed

1 sprig fresh rosemary

2 tablespoons butter (or canola oil)

1. Season both sides of the filets with ¼ teaspoon each of salt and pepper.

2. Preheat the oven to 400°F.

3. In a small bowl, start making the glaze by mashing the blueberries. Once mashed, add the wine, honey, lemon juice and rind, brown sugar, rosemary, and the remaining ¼ teaspoon of salt and pepper. Stir until combined. Set aside.

4. Heat a cast iron skillet over high heat, and once very hot, add the butter. Sear the filets in the skillet for 3 minutes. While the steak is searing, spoon the butter on top of the filets. Flip the filets and sear for an additional 3 minutes and continue spooning the butter over the steaks. Once both sides are seared, transfer your skillet directly to the oven for 4 to 7 minutes.

5. Meanwhile, heat a small saucepan over medium heat. Add the blueberry sauce and cook for 7 to 9 minutes or until the consistency becomes thick and syrupy.

6. Remove the filets from the skillet and set on plates. Let the filets rest for at least 5 minutes before serving.

7. Serve each filet topped with the blueberry sauce.

    Preparation tip: When cooking beef, it's important your meat gets to rest the same amount of time it cooked before slicing. Doing so ensures the meat will be juicier and taste better.

    Per serving: Calories: 471; Total fat: 23g; Total carbs: 17g; Fiber: 1g; Sugar: 15g; Protein: 38g; Sodium: 334mg

Pork Sliders

Prep time: 5 minutes / Cook time: 20 minutes, plus 30 minutes to marinate the slaw / Serves: 12

NUT-FREE, ONE POT, QUICK-PREP

These sliders are flavorful, tender, a little spicy, and very delicious! The marinated pulled pork and creamy coleslaw are a great combination of flavors that will invigorate your senses.

2½ pounds pork tenderloin

3¼ teaspoons sea salt, divided

1¼ teaspoons freshly ground black pepper

¼ cup mayonnaise

¼ teaspoon caraway seeds

1½ cups apple cider vinegar, plus 3 tablespoons, divided

4 tablespoons packed brown sugar, divided

1 cup shredded green (common) cabbage

1 cup shredded red cabbage

1 cup shredded carrots

2 tablespoons butter

1 tablespoon Garlic-Infused Oil (page 134)

½ teaspoon sriracha

2 tablespoons tomato paste

1 tablespoon Dijon mustard

1 cup Fody™ Low-FODMAP Barbeque Sauce

12 Udi's® Classic French Dinner Rolls (or low-FODMAP rolls or bread)

1. Take the pork out of the refrigerator at least 15 to 20 minutes before you begin cooking. Pat it dry with paper towels and season with 3 teaspoons of salt and the pepper.

2. In a medium bowl, beat together the mayonnaise, caraway seeds, 3 tablespoons of vinegar, 2 tablespoons of brown sugar, and the remaining ¼ teaspoon of salt. Stir in the green and red cabbage and carrots. Cover and refrigerate for 30 minutes.

3. Preheat a skillet over medium heat and add the butter. Brown the pork tenderloin for about 2 minutes on each side, and then cover the skillet. Reduce the heat to medium-low and continue cooking for 20 minutes, flipping once. When the internal temperature of the tenderloin reads 145°F, move the tenderloin to a clean surface and shred it with two forks.

4. In a medium saucepan over medium heat, combine the remaining 1½ cups of vinegar, oil, sriracha, brown sugar, tomato paste, Dijon mustard, and barbeque sauce. Cook for 5 minutes.

5. Add the shredded tenderloin to the saucepan and stir well to combine. While still hot, serve the pulled pork on buns topped with coleslaw mix.

Preparation tip: The vinegar helps further marinate and cook the pork. Make sure to coat all the pork with sauce, and if possible, let the sauce and pork sit for a few minutes.

Per serving: Calories: 289; Total fat: 10g; Total carbs: 30g; Fiber: 2g; Sugar: 11g; Protein: 20g; Sodium: 465mg

Pineapple Salsa Pork Chops

Prep time: 1 minute / Cook time: 10 minutes / Serves: 4

NUT-FREE, ONE POT, QUICK-PREP, UNDER 20 MINUTES

This super-easy recipe is great for a busy weeknight! The pork chops cook very fast and come out nice and tender with a sweet and spicy kick from the pineapple and salsa.

4 (5-ounce) boneless pork loin chops

¼ teaspoon kosher salt

¼ teaspoon freshly ground black pepper

1 tablespoon canola oil

1 (8-ounce) can unsweetened crushed pineapple, undrained

1 cup Casa de Sante Low-FODMAP Certified Salsa

2 tablespoons chopped fresh cilantro

1. Season the pork chops with the salt and pepper. Heat a large skillet over medium heat and add the canola oil; cook the pork chops for 2 to 3 minutes on the first side. Flip and cook until the pork chops are golden brown on the other side, 1 to 2 minutes more. Remove the pork chops from the skillet, and put them on a plate.

2. Using a paper towel, carefully wipe out the skillet and then add the canned pineapple and low-FODMAP salsa. Bring to a boil. Return the pork chops to the pan. Reduce the heat to low and simmer for 5 minutes, or until the pork is tender. Sprinkle with the cilantro and serve.

Shopping tip: When you create your grocery list, don't forget to also shop online. Some staples that are harder to find in stores, like Casa de Sante Low-FODMAP Certified Salsa, are great to have on hand for this recipe and others.

Per serving: Calories: 251; Total fat: 9g; Total carbs: 10g; Fiber: 1g; Sugar: 8g; Protein: 32g; Sodium: 324mg

Beef Broccoli Stir-Fry

Prep time: 5 minutes / Cook time: 20 minutes / Serves: 3

NUT-FREE, ONE POT, QUICK-PREP, UNDER 30 MINUTES

Beef and broccoli from your local Chinese restaurant likely contains garlic; however, you can very easily make your own at home. There may be no garlic in this dish, but it's very flavorful!

3 tablespoons cornstarch, divided

2 tablespoons plus ½ cup water, divided

1 pound flank steak, cut into thin 2-inch strips

¼ cup soy sauce

2 tablespoons brown sugar

¼ teaspoon red pepper flakes

1 tablespoon honey

1½ teaspoons diced fresh ginger

2 tablespoons vegetable oil, divided

½ cup water chestnuts, sliced

2 cups broccoli florets

1 medium red bell pepper, cored and sliced thin

½ to 1 tablespoon toasted sesame seeds, for serving

2 cups cooked rice, reheated

1. In a medium bowl, mix 2 tablespoons each of the cornstarch and water; toss with the beef.

2. In a small bowl, mix the soy sauce, brown sugar, red pepper flakes, honey, ginger, and the remaining 1 tablespoon of cornstarch and ½ cup of water until combined.

3. In a large skillet, heat 1 tablespoon of oil over medium-high heat; stir-fry the beef until browned, 4 to 6 minutes. Remove the steak from the pan.

4. In the same pan, stir-fry the water chestnuts, broccoli, and bell pepper in the remaining 1 tablespoon of oil over medium-high heat for 7 to 9 minutes. Whisk the soy sauce mixture again and add it to the pan. Cook and stir until thickened and coating the vegetables, about 4 minutes. Return the beef to the pan and stir until coated and heated through. Sprinkle with the sesame seeds and serve with the rice.

Preparation tip: If you prefer to use chicken, go right ahead! You'll need 1 pound of boneless skinless chicken breast cut into 1-inch pieces. Fourteen ounces of firm tofu also works well as long as you drain it beforehand (see my tofu draining tip on page 71).

Per serving: Calories: 569; Total fat: 11g; Total carbs: 75g; Fiber: 5g; Sugar: 16g; Protein: 42g; Sodium: 1331mg

Easy Shepherd's Pie

Prep time: 5 minutes / Cook time: 20 minutes / Serves: 6

NUT-FREE, QUICK-PREP, UNDER 30 MINUTES

No one will believe this delicious and hearty dish is from an elimination diet! You'll love the taste of this low-FODMAP shepherd's pie.

1 tablespoon olive oil

1 medium carrot, peeled and cut into thin rounds

1 pound 90% lean ground beef

¾ teaspoon dried rosemary

¾ teaspoon dried sage

½ teaspoon dried thyme

½ teaspoon kosher salt, divided

½ teaspoon freshly ground black pepper, divided

1 tablespoon Worcestershire sauce

2 tablespoons gluten-free low-FODMAP all-purpose flour

2 tablespoons tomato paste

1 cup low-FODMAP beef broth

½ cup frozen green beans

⅔ cup canned creamed corn

2 pounds russet potatoes, peeled, boiled, and mashed

8 tablespoons (1 stick) unsalted butter

¼ cup shredded Parmesan cheese (optional)

1. Heat the oil in a large skillet over medium-high heat. Add the carrot and cook for 3 minutes, stirring.

2. Add the ground beef, rosemary, sage, thyme, ¼ teaspoon of salt, and ¼ teaspoon of pepper. Stir well. Cook for 6 to 8 minutes, until the meat is browned.

3. Add the Worcestershire sauce and stir to combine. Cook for 1 minute.

4. Add the flour and tomato paste and stir to coat the meat. Add the broth, frozen green beans, and creamed corn. Stir well to combine. Bring to a boil then reduce the heat to simmer for 5 minutes, stirring occasionally.

5. Meanwhile, preheat the broiler.

6. In a medium bowl, combine the potatoes, butter, remaining ¼ teaspoon of salt, and remaining ¼ teaspoon of pepper. Reheat in the microwave for 2 minutes. Add the Parmesan cheese (if using) and stir.

7. Pour the meat mixture evenly into a 9-by-9-inch baking dish. Spread an even layer of the mashed potatoes over the meat.

8. Broil 4 to 6 inches away from the heat for 5 to 6 minutes or until the top is golden brown. Serve immediately.

Make-ahead tip: Make the mashed potatoes ahead of time with the butter, salt, and pepper and store in the refrigerator, covered.

Per serving: Calories: 474; Total fat: 27g; Total carbs: 35g; Fiber: 5g; Sugar: 5g; Protein: 25g; Sodium: 314mg

Beef, Bean, and Spinach Soup

Prep time: 5 minutes / **Cook time:** 25 minutes / **Serves:** 8 (Makes 2½ quarts)

NUT-FREE, ONE POT, QUICK-PREP

This hearty soup is delicious for a cold day or when you need something filling. Most beans are high-FODMAP; however, butter beans are low-FODMAP at ¼ cup per serving and a great option to add more variety into your diet.

1 pound lean ground beef

4 cups low-FODMAP broth

2 (14.5-ounce) cans unsalted diced tomatoes

¼ cup white cooking wine

1 cup canned butter beans, drained and rinsed

1 teaspoon dried basil

½ teaspoon dried oregano

¼ teaspoon kosher salt

½ teaspoon freshly ground black pepper

3 cups uncooked gluten-free low-FODMAP bow tie pasta

4 cups fresh spinach, coarsely chopped

8 ounces grated Parmesan cheese, divided

1. In a 6-quart stockpot over medium heat, cook the ground beef until it's no longer pink, 6 to 8 minutes; drain.
2. Stir in the broth, tomatoes, wine, beans, basil, oregano, salt, and pepper; bring to a boil. Stir in the pasta; return to a boil. Cook, uncovered, until the pasta is tender, 7 to 9 minutes.
3. Stir in the spinach and cook until wilted. Divide the soup among 8 bowls and top with the Parmesan cheese.

FODMAP tip: *When buying canned tomatoes make sure no high-FODMAP ingredients are present.*

Per serving: Calories: 381; Total fat: 16g; Total carbs: 28g; Fiber: 3g; Sugar: 4g; Protein: 30g; Sodium: 530mg

Corn Couscous and Chicken

Prep time: 10 minutes / Cook time: 15 minutes / Serves: 4

DAIRY-FREE, NUT-FREE, UNDER 30 MINUTES

This is a great recipe to get in some extra veggies. For veggie combinations, check your app; if two veggies become high in the same FODMAP group, stick to a full serving of one and a half serving of the other.

2 cups low-FODMAP vegetable stock

1 cup gluten-free corn couscous

4 chicken thighs

¼ teaspoon kosher salt

2 teaspoons ground sumac

2 teaspoons ground cumin

1 tablespoon Garlic-Infused Oil (page 134)

1 zucchini, sliced

1 cup broccoli florets

1 red bell pepper, diced

1 carrot, diced

½ cup diced pumpkin

8 ounces cherry tomatoes

1½ ounces sugar snap peas

2 cups baby spinach

1 tablespoon freshly squeezed lemon juice

2 tablespoons Garlic-Infused Oil (page 134)

1 teaspoon freshly ground black pepper

¼ cup chopped fresh parsley

¼ cup kalamata olives

2 tablespoons capers

1. In a large pot, bring the vegetable stock to a boil. Add the couscous. Turn off the heat, cover, and let stand.

2. Pat the chicken dry with a paper towel and season with the salt. Combine the sumac and cumin in a bowl and coat the chicken. Heat the oil in a pan, and cook the chicken for 7 to 8 minutes on each side until golden and cooked through. Remove the chicken from the pan and set aside.

3. Put the zucchini, broccoli florets, bell pepper, carrot, pumpkin, and tomatoes in the hot pan and cook, stirring for a few minutes. Add the sugar snap peas and spinach. Cook for another 2 to 3 minutes until the spinach wilts.

4. In a large mixing bowl, whisk together the lemon juice, oil, pepper, and parsley. Stir in the olives and capers.

5. Toss the couscous, veggies, and dressing in a bowl and top with the chicken.

Ingredient tip: Most couscous is made of durum wheat semolina, while corn couscous is made out of 100% maize (corn), which is low-FODMAP and gluten-free. You may also find other types of wheat-free couscous made from potato starch.

Per serving: Calories: 576; Total fat: 32g; Total carbs: 49g; Fiber: 8g; Sugar: 8g; Protein: 28g; Sodium: 641mg

One Pot Chicken Cordon Bleu

Prep time: 5 minutes / Cook time: 10 minutes / Serves: 4

NUT-FREE, ONE POT, QUICK-PREP, UNDER 20 MINUTES

Chicken cordon bleu has transformed over centuries. Several versions of this beloved dish exist that use different meats, cheeses, and preparation methods. For a recipe that may seem fancy, this low-FODMAP version is easy to make, plus it's ready in 15 minutes!

4 (6- to 8-ounce) boneless, skinless chicken breasts

½ cup gluten-free low-FODMAP all-purpose flour

¼ teaspoon dried thyme

⅛ teaspoon kosher salt

¼ teaspoon freshly ground black pepper

4 tablespoons unsalted butter

2 ounces thinly sliced ham

3 ounces thinly sliced Swiss cheese

1 tablespoon chopped fresh parsley

2 cups steamed whole broccolini (optional), for serving

1. Place the chicken breasts on a cutting board, and with a meat mallet, pound each breast until flattened.

2. Put the flour in a wide, shallow dish, along with the thyme, salt, and pepper, and whisk to combine. Coat each breast in the flour mixture and shake off any excess.

3. Melt the butter in a large sauté pan or skillet over medium heat. When it foams, add the chicken breasts. Cook on one side until golden brown, about 4 minutes. Flip the chicken breasts and place 1 slice of ham and 1 slice of Swiss cheese on each breast. Cover the pot and cook for another 4 minutes or until the breasts are cooked through.

4. Garnish with the parsley and serve with the steamed broccolini (if using).

   Serving tip: This dish also pairs well with sautéed green beans, steamed spinach, rice, low-FODMAP pasta, or polenta.

   Per serving: Calories: 437; Total fat: 21g; Total carbs: 13g; Fiber: 2g; Sugar: 0g; Protein: 49g; Sodium: 412mg

Ground Beef, Rice, and Veggie Bake

Prep time: 5 minutes / Cook time: 25 minutes / Serves: 4

NUT-FREE, ONE POT, QUICK-PREP

One pan, four servings of veggies, and you have a delicious meal on the table in half an hour. This filling and nutritious dish is packed with flavor!

1 tablespoon Garlic-Infused Oil (page 134)

1 pound ground beef

1 medium carrot, diced

1 medium zucchini, diced

1 medium red bell pepper, diced

1 cup diced eggplant

1 cup sliced leeks, green parts only

7½ inch (20-cm) celery stalk, diced

16 ounces low-FODMAP beef stock

1 (14-ounce) can diced tomatoes

2 heaped teaspoons seeded mustard

2 tablespoons tomato paste

4 ounces Worcestershire sauce

2 cups cooked rice

Kosher salt

Freshly ground black pepper

2 cups grated cheese

1. Heat the oil in a large oven-safe skillet and brown the ground beef. Set the beef aside.

2. Combine the carrot, zucchini, bell pepper, eggplant, leeks, and celery in the pan. Cook, stirring, for 5 minutes until the vegetables begin to soften.

3. Return the beef to the skillet and add the beef stock, tomatoes, mustard, tomato paste, Worcestershire sauce, and cooked rice. Reduce the heat to low and simmer for 20 minutes. Season with salt and pepper to taste.

4. Top with the grated cheese and place under a hot broiler for 5 minutes or until golden.

FODMAP tip: *One low-FODMAP serving of celery is equal to one-quarter of a stalk. When buying canned tomatoes be sure that no high-FODMAP ingredients are present.*

Per serving: Calories: 694; Total fat: 31g; Total carbs: 60g; Fiber: 5g; Sugar: 15g; Protein: 44g; Sodium: 1065mg

Chicken and Corn Soup

Prep time: 5 minutes / Cook time: 20 minutes / Serves: 5

DAIRY-FREE, NUT-FREE, QUICK-PREP, UNDER 30 MINUTES

This Chicken and Corn Soup is the perfect comfort food to share with friends or just to warm you up when it's cold outside. This delicious recipe is a great example of how good low-FODMAP nutrition can also be about comfort, warmth, pleasure, friends, and celebration.

32 ounces low-FODMAP chicken stock

1 (14-ounce) can creamed corn

1 (6-ounce) can coconut milk

1 zucchini, diced

1 carrot, diced

1 teaspoon fish sauce

4 chicken thighs

Kosher salt

Freshly ground black pepper

1 tablespoon Garlic-Infused Oil (page 134)

2 tablespoons chopped fresh coriander leaves

2 tablespoons chopped green scallion leaves

1. Put the chicken stock, creamed corn, coconut milk, zucchini, carrot, and fish sauce in a large pot and bring to a boil. Reduce the heat and simmer.

2. Meanwhile, season the chicken thighs with salt and pepper. Heat the oil in a large pan and cook the chicken thighs for 5 minutes on each side until almost cooked through.

3. Once the chicken is cooled, dice finely and add to the stock mixture. Simmer for another 5 minutes until the chicken is cooked through. Serve with the coriander and scallion leaves.

Preparation tip: Feeling hungry? Serve each portion over ½ cup of cooked brown rice.

Per serving: Calories: 379; Total fat: 12g; Total carbs: 16g; Fiber: 2g; Sugar: 8g; Protein: 19g; Sodium: 451mg

Chicken Veggie Parmesan Sandwiches

Prep time: 5 minutes / **Cook time:** 15 minutes / **Serves:** 4

NUT-FREE, ONE POT, QUICK-PREP, UNDER 30 MINUTES

Chicken Parmesan sandwiches from Italian restaurants are a classic in New York, where I grew up. They are well loved by many and for good reason—they taste out of this world. My recipe is free of many of the FODMAPs found in chicken Parmesan sandwiches but still tastes authentic.

1 cup gluten-free low-FODMAP all-purpose flour

2 large eggs, lightly beaten

1½ cups gluten-free plain bread crumbs

½ cup grated Parmesan cheese

4 (5-ounce) boneless skinless chicken breast halves

¼ teaspoon kosher salt

¼ teaspoon freshly ground black pepper

1 tablespoon butter

8 cups baby spinach

1 (6.5-ounce) can sliced mushrooms, drained

Nonstick cooking spray

4 gluten-free low-FODMAP dinner rolls

4 slices mozzarella cheese

½ cup low-FODMAP marinara sauce, warmed

1. Put the flour and eggs in separate shallow bowls.
2. In another shallow bowl, toss the bread crumbs with the Parmesan cheese.
3. Pound the chicken with a meat mallet to ½-inch thickness; sprinkle with the salt and pepper.
4. Dip the chicken in the flour to lightly coat both sides. Dip in the egg, then in the crumb mixture.
5. In a large skillet, heat the butter over medium heat. Once the butter is halfway melted, add the spinach and sliced mushrooms. Cook until the spinach is wilted then set aside in a bowl and cover with aluminum foil.
6. Spray the same skillet with nonstick cooking spray and add the chicken; cook until golden brown, 4 to 5 minutes per side.
7. Serve the chicken Parmesan on rolls with the spinach and mushrooms, 1 slice of mozzarella cheese and 1 to 2 tablespoons of marinara sauce.

FODMAP tip: Not all mushrooms are high-FODMAP! Presently, canned champignon mushrooms or other canned mushrooms (packed in water and salt), fresh oyster mushrooms, and small amounts of dried porcini mushrooms are low-FODMAP.

Per serving: Calories: 661; Total fat: 18g; Total carbs: 69g; Fiber: 9g; Sugar: 5g; Protein: 57g; Sodium: 943mg

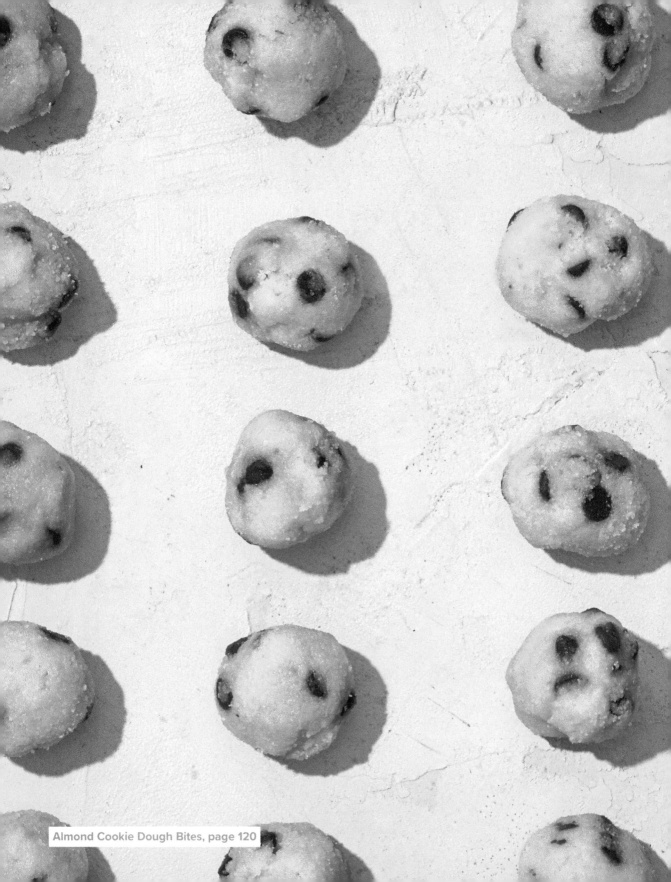

Almond Cookie Dough Bites, page 120

CHAPTER 7

Snacks and Desserts

Fruit and Cheese Kebabs

Prep time: 2 minutes / Serves: 2

5 INGREDIENTS OR LESS, NUT-FREE, VEGETARIAN, QUICK-PREP, UNDER 10 MINUTES

For a healthy and filling low-FODMAP treat, these Fruit and Cheese Kebabs are just the trick. You can always get creative and try different cheese or fruit combinations, but the recipe below is my go-to for delectable kebabs.

**8 kiwi slices from
2 peeled kiwis**

8 fresh raspberries

8 cubes cheddar cheese

On a skewer, alternate slices of kiwi, raspberries, and cheese. Repeat with the other skewer.

Ingredient tip: Try different low-FODMAP cheeses: Havarti, Swiss, mozzarella, Monterey Jack, and Colby are great examples. A variation I like is 10 blueberries, 5 medium strawberries, and 4 cubes of cheddar cheese.

Per serving: Calories: 326; Total fat: 23g; Total carbs: 21g; Fiber: 7g; Sugar: 11g; Protein: 19g; Sodium: 425mg

Goat Cheese Dip

Prep time: 5 minutes / Makes: about 1½ cups

NUT-FREE, QUICK-PREP, UNDER 10 MINUTES

If you like goat cheese, you will love this dip. Tangy and creamy, this dip is great for your next gathering or as a crudité with low-FODMAP vegetables.

8 ounces plain goat cheese

3 tablespoons cream cheese

¼ cup water chestnuts, sliced

1 ounce baby spinach

1 tablespoon chopped scallions, green parts only

⅛ teaspoon wheat-free asafetida powder (optional)

¼ teaspoon cayenne pepper

2 tablespoons extra-virgin olive oil

¼ teaspoon kosher salt, plus more for seasoning

¼ teaspoon freshly ground black pepper, plus more for seasoning

1. Combine the goat cheese, cream cheese, water chestnuts, spinach, scallions, asafetida powder (if using), cayenne pepper, oil, salt, and pepper in a food processor. Pulse until smooth and the spinach is completely blended and the dip is emerald green. Stop pulsing along the way and scrape down the sides with a spatula if needed.

2. Add more salt and pepper as desired. Serve immediately with gluten-free and low-FODMAP pita chips, or low-FODMAP fresh vegetables.

Ingredient tip: Two tablespoons of regular cream cheese is equal to 1 low-FODMAP serving. Anything more becomes moderate- to high-FODMAP. Lactose-free cream cheese is also an alternative and can be consumed in larger quantities.

Storage tip: Store leftovers in an airtight container in the refrigerator for up to 4 days.

Per serving (2 tablespoons): Calories: 80; Total fat: 7g; Total carbs: 1g; Fiber: 0g; Sugar: 0g; Protein: 4g; Sodium: 104mg

Cream Cheese and Ham Pinwheels

Prep time: 5 minutes, plus 1 hour to chill / Serves: 8

5 INGREDIENTS OR LESS, NUT-FREE, QUICK-PREP, UNDER 10 MINUTES

These pinwheels are great snacks or party appetizers. Green Valley Creamery™ offers delicious lactose-free cream cheese and sour cream that can be used in this recipe. If your local grocer doesn't carry lactose-free cream cheese, sour cream, yogurt, or kefir, ask the manager to put in a special order for you. Don't be shy—this recipe is worth it!

8 ounces lactose-free cream cheese

4 ounces diced ham

2 tablespoons low-FODMAP salsa

1 tablespoon lactose-free sour cream

8 soft corn tortillas

1. Put the cream cheese in a food processor and pulse a few times to get a smooth consistency. Add the ham and pulse until well mixed with the cream cheese. Add the salsa and sour cream and pulse until the entire mixture is pink.

2. Spread the mixture evenly over each tortilla. Roll up tightly and wrap in plastic. Refrigerate until firm, about 1 hour. Unwrap and cut into ¾-inch pinwheels.

Ingredient tip: When you go to the deli counter at your local grocer, ask the attendant to show you the ingredients to make sure the ham was not made with high-FODMAPs.

Per serving: Calories: 178; Total fat: 12g; Total carbs: 12g; Fiber: 2g; Sugar: 0g; Protein: 6g; Sodium: 304mg

Candied Pecans

Prep time: 2 minutes / Cook time: 4 minutes / Serves: 4

5 INGREDIENTS OR LESS, VEGAN, QUICK-PREP, UNDER 10 MINUTES

These Candied Pecans are a super easy low-FODMAP treat. Try them as a snack, throw them in a greens or grains salad, use as a topping in the Bacon Pecan Quinoa Salad (page 48), or incorporate them into baking recipes such as the Sweet Potato Chocolate Pancakes (page 31).

1½ tablespoons packed brown sugar

1½ teaspoons water

⅛ teaspoon pure vanilla extract

⅛ teaspoon kosher salt

1 cup pecan halves

1. In a small bowl, combine the brown sugar, water, vanilla, and salt; stir to combine.

2. In a medium-large saucepan over medium heat, toast the pecans for about 3 minutes, stirring occasionally.

3. Using a rubber spatula, quickly scoop out the brown sugar mixture into the pan with the pecans. Stir continuously for 15 to 20 seconds, until the pecans are thoroughly coated. Immediately remove from the heat.

4. Spread the pecans on a piece of parchment paper to cool.

FODMAP tip: *One low-FODMAP serving of pecans is equal to 10 halves or 20 grams.*

Storage tip: Store the pecans in an airtight container for up to a week.

Per serving: Calories: 208; Total fat: 20g; Total carbs: 7g; Fiber: 3g; Sugar: 4g; Protein: 3g; Sodium: 17mg

Warm Banana Roll-Up

Prep time: **3 minutes** / Cook time: **5 minutes** / Serves: **1**

NUT-FREE, QUICK-PREP, UNDER 10 MINUTES

Bananas and chocolate make a delicious and low-FODMAP combo! Make sure the banana is firm and yellow-light green, not deeper yellow with brown spots. This recipe calls for dark chocolate, but you can use 20 grams of milk or 25 grams of white chocolate if you prefer.

1 medium firm banana

1 gluten-free low-FODMAP wrap

⅛ teaspoon ground cinnamon

2 teaspoons maple syrup

1 ounce dark mini chocolate chips

⅔ scoop vanilla ice cream (optional)

1. Preheat the oven's broiler. Line a baking sheet with aluminum foil.

2. Slice the banana into coins. Put the banana on the wrap. Place the wrap on the prepared baking sheet. Sprinkle the cinnamon and drizzle the maple syrup evenly over the banana. Sprinkle evenly with the chocolate chips.

3. Put the baking sheet under the broiler for 1 to 3 minutes or until the chocolate is melted. Roll up and eat with vanilla ice cream (if using).

Ingredient tip: A 30-gram scoop of vanilla ice cream is low-FODMAP. Be sure the ice cream you buy does not contain high-FODMAP ingredients.

Per serving: Calories: 346; Total fat: 12g; Total carbs: 62g; Fiber: 4g; Sugar: 32g; Protein: 6g; Sodium: 192mg

Fruit and Chocolate Popcorn Snack Mix

Prep time: 3 minutes / Cook time: 5 minutes / Serves: 1 (Makes 5 cups)

5 INGREDIENTS OR LESS, QUICK-PREP, UNDER 10 MINUTES

Popcorn is a tasty low-FODMAP snack and a great source of fiber! Be sure to stick to natural or plain popcorn; other packaged popcorns sometimes contain milk products, garlic or onion powder, or "natural flavors" that may contain high-FODMAPs.

⅓ **cup popcorn kernels**

1 tablespoon no sugar added cranberries

¾ **cup Kellogg's Original Crispix® cereal**

10 unsalted macadamia nuts

1 ounce dark chocolate morsels (optional)

1. Pour the popcorn kernels into a brown paper bag. Fold the top of the bag over tightly.

2. Cook in the microwave on full power for 2½ to 3 minutes or until you hear a pause of about 2 seconds between pops.

3. Combine the popcorn with the cranberries, cereal, macadamia nuts, and chocolate (if using) in a zip-top bag for easy, portable snacking.

   Make-ahead tip: Make a week's worth of these snack bags ahead of time to have on hand for your busy day.

   Ingredient tip: To change things up, add ½ cup of pretzels, 20 grams of milk chocolate, 25 grams of white chocolate, plain potato chips, other certi-fied low-FODMAP cereals, low-FODMAP nuts like 32 peanuts, 10 almonds, or 20 grams of dried figs, 15 banana chips, or 3 teaspoons of goji berries. Just remember to stick to one serving of low-FODMAP fruit per bag.

   Per serving: Calories: 417; Total fat: 17g; Total carbs: 59g; Fiber: 8g; Sugar: 4g; Protein: 9g; Sodium: 213mg

Kiwi Yogurt Cups

Prep time: 5 minutes / Serves: 1

5 INGREDIENTS OR LESS, NUT-FREE, VEGETARIAN, QUICK-PREP, UNDER 10 MINUTES

This is a light, refreshing, and healthy snack that can also be dessert. Kiwis are a great natural source of fiber.

2 kiwi fruits

1 tablespoon maple syrup

1 teaspoon lemon zest

1 tablespoon pumpkin seeds, divided

1 small tub lactose-free vanilla yogurt

1. Peel and chop the kiwis and put them in a bowl with the maple syrup and lemon zest; stir and mix well.

2. In a glass mason jar or glass cup, alternate one layer of kiwi, pumpkin seeds, and yogurt. Alternate again until all the ingredients are used.

Substitution tip: Try using lime zest, a different low-FODMAP fruit, or hemp seeds for some variety.

Storage tip: Store the yogurt cup for up to 3 days in the refrigerator in a sealed mason jar or airtight container.

Per serving: Calories: 273; Total fat: 5g; Total carbs: 51g; Fiber: 5g; Sugar: 34g; Protein: 10g; Sodium: 98mg

Chocolate Tahini Fudge

Prep time: 10 minutes, plus 1 hour and 10 minutes for freezing /
Cook time: 1 minute / **Serves:** 20

DAIRY-FREE, VEGAN

Tahini is all the rage these days and for good reason. It tastes so good with many different recipes. This delectable Chocolate Tahini Fudge is low in sugar and easy to make; it's a quick-preparation that is made all the more delicious by freezing the fudge for about an hour, but it's worth the wait.

½ **cup refined coconut oil**

¾ **cup cocoa powder**

¾ **cup tahini paste**

⅓ **cup maple syrup**

1 **teaspoon pure vanilla extract**

⅛ **teaspoon Himalayan sea salt**

1. Line a 9-by-5-inch loaf pan with parchment paper.

2. Melt the coconut oil in the microwave for 30 seconds. Pour into a medium mixing bowl. Add the cocoa powder, tahini paste, maple syrup, vanilla extract, and salt. Whisk until completely smooth.

3. Pour the mixture into the prepared pan. Cover with plastic wrap or parchment paper and secure the covering with a rubber band so it doesn't touch the fudge mixture. Put it in the freezer until chilled and firm; 50 to 70 minutes.

4. Using a sharp knife, cut into 20 small squares and serve.

   Preparation tip: This recipe already has coconut oil in it so be sure to separate the tahini paste from the oil in the jar.

   Per serving: Calories: 122; Total fat: 11g; Total carbs: 7g; Fiber: 2g; Sugar: 3g; Protein: 2g; Sodium: 16mg

Vegan Chocolate Pudding with Sea Salt

Prep time: 2 minutes / Cook time: 5 minutes, plus 5 minutes to cool / Serves: 4

VEGAN, QUICK-PREP, UNDER 10 MINUTES

Making pudding at home is easy and such a fun treat. The velvety smooth chocolate in this recipe will make it an instant family favorite. Try topping with flaked sea salt, roughly chopped dark chocolate (1 ounce per serving), or non-vegan whipped cream (½ cup per serving).

1 can full-fat coconut milk

3 tablespoons cornstarch

2 tablespoons cocoa powder

⅓ cup lightly packed brown sugar

1 teaspoon pure vanilla extract

¼ teaspoon ground cinnamon

⅛ teaspoon sea salt

Flaked sea salt, for topping (optional)

1. Vigorously shake the can of coconut milk. In a medium bowl, whisk the coconut milk and cornstarch until no lumps remain.

2. Into a large saucepan over medium heat, pour the coconut milk mixture along with the cocoa powder, brown sugar, vanilla, cinnamon, and salt. Cook, whisking constantly, until boiling. Once thickened, remove from the heat.

3. Let cool for 5 minutes, and serve immediately with a pinch of flaked sea salt on top (if using).

Storage tip: Store the pudding in an airtight container in the refrigerator for up to 3 days.

Per serving: Calories: 346; Total fat: 26g; Total carbs: 31g; Fiber: 3g; Sugar: 22g; Protein: 3g; Sodium: 81mg

Chickpea Vegan Cookie Dough

Prep time: 1 minute / Cook time: 5 minutes / Serves: 5

5 INGREDIENTS OR LESS, VEGAN, QUICK-PREP, UNDER 10 MINUTES

Chickpeas are rich in plant-based protein and fiber, which will help keep you satisfied. So, why not reap the benefits of nutrients while having dessert? Serve this up to your family and friends and enjoy!

1¼ cups canned chickpeas, drained and rinsed

½ cup plus 2 tablespoons natural peanut butter

¼ cup maple syrup

⅛ teaspoon kosher salt or sea salt

½ cup vegan dark mini chocolate chips

1. Put the chickpeas in a food processor with the peanut butter, maple syrup, salt, and chocolate chips. Blend until mostly smooth but still contains some whole chocolate chips.

2. Divide the cookie dough among 5 bowls and serve.

> **FODMAP tip:** *One low-FODMAP serving of dark chocolate is equal to about 5 squares. When using canned chickpeas, always drain and rinse them before consuming. Canned chickpeas are okay to consume at ¼ cup per serving.*

Serving tip: This cookie dough tastes best when it's put in an airtight container and chilled in the refrigerator for 30 minutes or more before serving.

Per serving: Calories: 425; Total fat: 23g; Total carbs: 46g; Fiber: 5g; Sugar: 24g; Protein: 15g; Sodium: 245mg

Sweet and Spicy Baked Plantains

Prep time: 3 minutes / Cook time: 20 minutes / Serves: 6

DAIRY-FREE, NUT-FREE, VEGAN, QUICK-PREP, UNDER 30 MINUTES

While growing up in New York and visiting South American countries, I've tried many versions of fried plantains. They can be a bit heavy when fried, but baking them makes them less fatty and easier on the gut. You'll love this super easy and fiber-filled snack.

2 medium ripe plantains, peeled

¼ teaspoon chili powder

¼ teaspoon ground cinnamon

½ tablespoon packed brown sugar

2 tablespoons olive oil

¼ teaspoon kosher salt or sea salt

1. Preheat the oven to 425°F. Line a large baking sheet with parchment paper.

2. Slice the plantains at an angle into ¼-inch slices.

3. Put the plantain slices in a medium bowl and toss with the chili powder, cinnamon, brown sugar, olive oil, and salt.

4. Lay the plantains across the prepared baking sheet and bake for 10 minutes. Using a spatula, flip over the plantains and bake for another 10 minutes. Serve immediately or at room temperature.

Serving tip: Forgo the spice and sugar and just make the plantains with oil and salt.

Storage tip: Store leftovers in an airtight container at room temperature for 5 to 6 days.

Per serving: Calories: 116; Total fat: 5g; Total carbs: 20g; Fiber: 2g; Sugar: 10g; Protein: 1g; Sodium: 27mg

No Bake Chocolate Cheesecake

Prep time: 5 minutes / Cook time: 10 minutes, plus 3 hours to chill / Serves: 16

VEGETARIAN, QUICK-PREP, UNDER 20 MINUTES

Want to enjoy the decadence of cheesecake without all the added sugar? The melted chocolate mixed with the cream cheese really steals the show in this recipe. This family-approved dessert proves once again that you can eat low-FODMAP and not feel deprived of the foods and flavors you love.

For the crust

1⅔ cups almond flour

1 tablespoon plus ½ teaspoon Pyure® Organic Stevia packets

¾ teaspoon ground cinnamon

½ cup butter, melted

Nonstick cooking spray (optional)

For the filling

16 ounces lactose-free cream cheese, softened

¼ cup Pyure® Organic Stevia

2 tablespoons lactose-free milk

1 teaspoon pure vanilla extract

8 ounces dark chocolate baking bar

1. Whisk together the almond flour, stevia, and cinnamon in a medium bowl. When smooth, slowly whisk in the butter. Line a 9-inch springform pan with parchment paper or spray with nonstick cooking spray. Pat the mixture into the bottom of the pan, cover with plastic wrap, and put in the freezer.

2. In the bowl of a stand mixer, mix the cream cheese and stevia until smooth. Add the milk and vanilla, and mix again.

3. In a microwave-safe bowl, melt the chocolate in 30-second increments in the microwave, whisking once it starts to melt. Continue whisking until completely melted. Do not overcook as the chocolate can burn.

4. Add the melted chocolate to the stand mixer and mix until the cream cheese mixture turns brown. Use a spatula to scrape down the sides if necessary.

5. Remove the springform pan from the freezer. Pour the cream cheese mixture over the crust, using a spatula to smooth the top. Cover with plastic wrap and refrigerate for 2 to 3 hours. Leftovers can be refrigerated, covered, for up to 5 days.

Substitution tip: You can use 3 tablespoons of sugar in place of the stevia for the crust and ½ cup of sugar in place of the stevia for the filling.

Per serving: Calories: 279; Total fat: 25g; Total carbs: 13g; Fiber: 3g; Sugar: 4g; Protein: 5g; Sodium: 128mg

Almond Cookie Dough Bites

Prep time: 5 minutes, plus 20 minutes to chill / Makes: 20

VEGAN, QUICK-PREP, UNDER 30 MINUTES

I love storing these cookie dough bites in the freezer. They take only a couple minutes to thaw before you can enjoy them. Freezing treats is a great way to always have something scrumptious on hand.

2 cups almond flour

½ cup refined coconut oil, melted

⅓ cup vegan confectioners' sugar

2 tablespoons Pyure® Organic Stevia

½ teaspoon pure vanilla extract

½ teaspoon sea salt

⅔ cup vegan mini dark chocolate chips

1. In a medium bowl, combine the almond flour, coconut oil, confectioners' sugar, stevia, vanilla, and salt. Stir until thickened and the mixture forms into dough. Fold in the chocolate chips.

2. Using a cookie scoop or tablespoon, scoop and make 20 balls. Cover the bowl with plastic wrap and put in the refrigerator to firm slightly, 15 to 20 minutes.

Ingredient tip: If you do not have Pyure® Organic Stevia, use another brand of stevia powder (check for additional high-FODMAP Polyols) or ¼ cup of sugar.

Preparation tip: If you're concerned about consuming raw flour, spread the almond flour in an even layer on a baking sheet and bake for 5 minutes at 350°F before making this recipe.

Storage tip: Store in an airtight container in the refrigerator for up to 1 week or in the freezer for up to 1 month.

Per serving (1 dough bite): Calories: 120; Total fat: 10g; Total carbs: 8g; Fiber: 1g; Sugar: 2g; Protein: 2g; Sodium: 49mg

Coconut Macaroons

Prep time: 10 minutes / Cook time: 20 minutes, plus 1 hour to cool / Makes: 15

DAIRY-FREE, VEGETARIAN

Light and slightly crunchy, these simple macaroons make a great snack or dessert.

Nonstick cooking spray

2½ tablespoons
   coconut oil, melted

2 cups light
   shredded coconut

2 tablespoons rice flour

⅓ cup egg whites
   (2 egg whites)

¼ cup granulated
   cane sugar

1 teaspoon pure
   vanilla extract

⅛ teaspoon sea salt

½ tablespoon organic
   maple syrup

1. Preheat the oven to 350°F. Lightly spray a nonstick baking sheet with the nonstick cooking spray.

2. Mix the melted coconut oil, coconut shreds, and rice flour on high speed in a stand mixer.

3. In a separate bowl, whisk together the egg whites, sugar, vanilla, and salt.

4. Combine the two mixtures and mix on high speed for 30 to 45 seconds. Add the maple syrup and mix again until fully combined.

5. Shape the mixture into 15 (1-inch) balls and put them on the prepared baking sheet. Bake at 350° for 15 to 20 minutes. Remove from the oven and allow to cool for 30 minutes to an hour.

Preparation tip: Try adding a fine drizzle of melted dark chocolate to the tops of the macaroons or lightly sprinkle with cinnamon and confectioners' sugar.

Per serving: Calories: 224; Total fat: 10g; Total carbs: 8g; Fiber: 2g; Sugar: 4g; Protein: 1g; Sodium: 25mg

Raisin Sunflower Coconut Oat Bars

Prep time: 5 minutes / Cook time: 30 minutes / Makes: 18

VEGAN, QUICK-PREP

These Raisin Sunflower Coconut Oat Bars will give you energy and fill you up, no matter where the day takes you. There's no need to stand in the grocery store reading labels to decipher which bars are high-FODMAP. Now you can easily make your own oat bars at home!

Nonstick cooking spray (optional)

2 cups quick cooking oats

⅔ cup unsweetened flaked coconut

2 cups gluten-free low-FODMAP all-purpose flour

1½ cups lightly packed brown sugar

1 teaspoon baking soda

1 teaspoon sea salt

1 teaspoon pure vanilla extract

2 Flax Eggs (page 143)

1¼ cups Nutiva Organic Vegan Shortening, melted

⅓ cup sunflower seeds

⅔ cup raisins

1. Preheat the oven to 350°F. Line a 12-by-9-inch baking dish with parchment paper or spray the pan with nonstick cooking spray.

2. Put the oats, coconut, flour, brown sugar, baking soda, sea salt, vanilla, flax eggs, and shortening in a large mixing bowl and stir until just combined. Fold in the sunflower seeds and raisins.

3. Spread the oat mixture onto the prepared baking dish. Bake for 25 to 30 minutes or until a fork or toothpick comes out partially clean.

4. Let cool for 1 hour, then cut into 18 bars and wrap each bar individually in plastic wrap.

Substitution tip: To make this recipe non-vegan, use 1¼ cups of melted butter in place of the vegan shortening and 2 regular eggs instead of the Flax Eggs.

Storage tip: Store in the refrigerator for 5 days or in a zip-top bag in the freezer for up to 4 months.

Per serving: Calories: 312; Total fat: 18g; Total carbs: 35g; Fiber: 3g; Sugar: 15g; Protein: 3g; Sodium: 182mg

Cranberry Scones with Lemon Glaze

Prep time: 10 minutes / Cook time: 20 minutes / Serves: 6

NUT-FREE, VEGETARIAN

There's nothing like the sweet smell of scones and a cup of low-FODMAP tea first thing in the morning. These scones are a family favorite, and I also love to make them when we have company over. If you don't have a lemon, use an orange for the zest and juice. Lactose-free full-fat milk is best, but unsweetened almond milk works well too. Enjoy!

For the scones

1¾ cups gluten-free low-FODMAP all-purpose flour

¼ cup cornstarch

2 teaspoons baking powder

¼ teaspoon baking soda

½ teaspoon kosher salt

2 teaspoons granulated sugar

Zest of 1 medium lemon

5 tablespoons unsalted butter, chopped into small chunks and chilled

½ cup dried cranberries

¾ cup lactose-free full-fat milk, plus 2 tablespoons

1 tablespoon freshly squeezed lemon juice

2 tablespoons maple syrup

For the glaze

1 cup powdered sugar

2 tablespoons freshly squeezed lemon juice, or more

1. Preheat the oven to 400°F. Line a rimmed baking sheet with parchment paper.

2. In a large bowl, sift and combine the flour, cornstarch, baking powder, baking soda, salt, granulated sugar, and lemon zest, and whisk well.

3. Add the butter, and toss with the dry ingredients. Massage every piece of butter between your fingers, flattening the pieces. Add the cranberries, and toss to combine.

4. Create a well in the center of the dry ingredients and add ¾ cup of milk, lemon juice, and maple syrup. Mix gently until the dough is the same consistency throughout. If necessary, dust your hands with flour to keep from sticking.

5. Lay a large piece of plastic wrap on a clean countertop and place the dough in the middle. Press down to make a disk that's about 7 inches in diameter. Dust lightly with more flour before wrapping the disk tightly in the plastic wrap. Put the dough in the freezer to chill for 10 minutes.

6. Remove the dough from the freezer and unwrap it. Dust a butter knife with flour and cut the dough into 2 equal halves, then cut each of those halves into 3 equal triangles. Place the wedges on the prepared baking sheet, leaving 2 inches between each piece. Brush the tops of the scones with the remaining 2 tablespoons of milk. Sprinkle the tops generously with granulated sugar.

Continued ▶

Cranberry Scones with Lemon Glaze
continued

7. Put the baking sheet in the center of the preheated oven and bake for 20 minutes.

8. Meanwhile, whisk the powdered sugar and lemon juice together in a small bowl to make the glaze.

9. When the scones are done baking, they should be puffed and golden on the edges. Remove the scones from the oven and let cool for 10 minutes on the baking sheet before drizzling the glaze over the scones. Allow the glaze to set before serving.

Ingredient tip: I recommend using Better Batter All Purpose Flour Mix; different flour brands can yield different results for this recipe. If you use a low-FODMAP all-purpose flour that doesn't contain xanthan gum, add 1 teaspoon of xanthan gum to the flour.

Preparation tip: Be sure to sift your flour well beforehand and use a spoon to drop the flour into your measuring cup. If you don't have a flour sifter, a mesh strainer will work well too.

Per serving: Calories: 403; Total fat: 11g; Total carbs: 72g; Fiber: 5g; Sugar: 36g; Protein: 5g; Sodium: 190mg

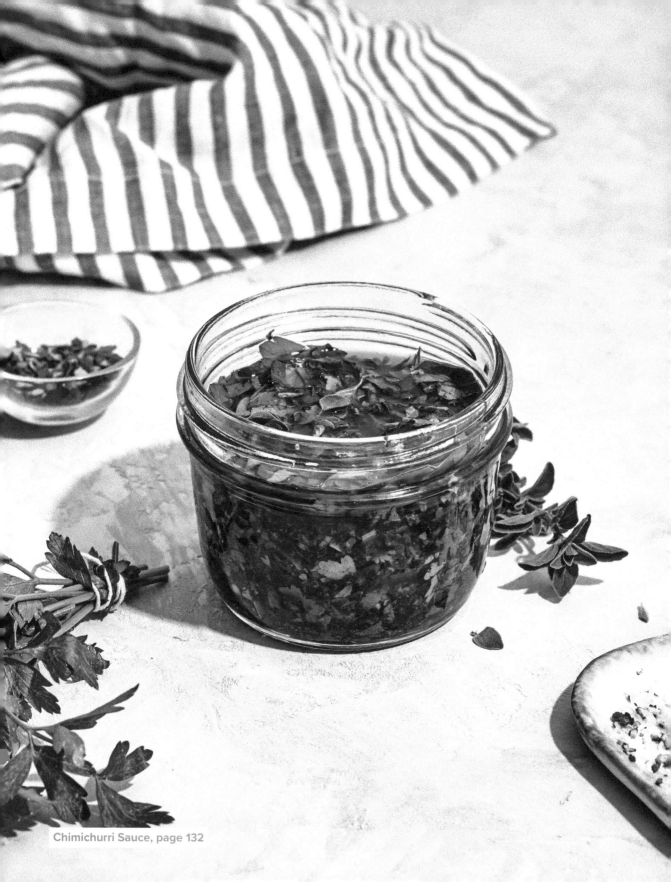

Chimichurri Sauce, page 132

CHAPTER 8

Broths, Sauces, Oils, and Dressings

Vegetable Herb Broth

Prep time: 5 minutes / Cook time: 20+ minutes / Makes: 4 quarts

NUT-FREE, VEGAN, QUICK-PREP

This broth is a delicious and good low-FODMAP alternative to store-bought broths. Instead of garlic or onion, leek leaves are used for an "oniony" flavor. Use this broth as the base for your next soup, add it to mashed potatoes for a savory flavor, incorporate it in a vegetable risotto dish, or use it to cook rice, quinoa, or polenta instead of using plain old water.

4 quarts water

2 medium carrots, peeled and roughly diced

½ celery stalk, roughly diced

2 leek leaves, chopped

3 sprigs (2 teaspoons) fresh parsley

4 sprigs fresh thyme

1 dried bay leaf

¼ teaspoon kosher salt

½ teaspoon peppercorns

1. Fill a large pot with the water, carrots, celery, leek leaves, parsley, thyme, bay leaf, salt, and peppercorns.

2. Bring to a low boil over high heat, and then reduce to a simmer and let cook for at least 20 minutes and up to 40. Strain and use immediately.

Storage tip: Store in an airtight container in the refrigerator for 4 to 5 days, or store in the freezer for 3 to 4 months.

Per serving (1 cup): Calories: 20; Total fat: 0g; Total carbs: 4g; Fiber: 1g; Sugar: 3g; Protein: 1g; Sodium: 140mg

Chicken Stock

Prep time: 5 minutes / Cook time: 30+ minutes / Makes: 4 quarts

NUT-FREE, QUICK-PREP

One of the most versatile staples in a low-FODMAP kitchen is low-FODMAP chicken stock. Unless you have access to certified low-FODMAP stock, you'll find that many other vegetable, chicken, or beef stocks contain high-FODMAPs that can be bothersome to the gut. Enjoy this recipe in my One Pot Creamy Mexican Mac 'n' Cheese (page 92) or Easy Shepherd's Pie (page 98).

4 quarts water

Chicken bones from 1 large chicken

2 large carrots, peeled and roughly diced

½ celery stalk, roughly diced

1 sprig fresh oregano

3 sprigs fresh parsley

3 sprigs fresh thyme

2 dried bay leaves

½ teaspoon peppercorns

¼ teaspoon kosher salt

1. Fill a large pot with the water and add the chicken bones, carrots, celery, oregano, parsley, thyme, bay leaves, peppercorns, and salt. Bring to a low boil over high heat, then reduce to a simmer and let cook for 30 minutes or as much as 1 hour.

2. Strain and use immediately.

Storage tip: Store in an airtight container in the refrigerator for 4 to 5 days, or store in the freezer for 3 to 4 months.

Per serving (1 cup): Calories: 29; Total fat: 0g; Total carbs: 3g; Fiber: 0g; Sugar: 1g; Protein: 4g; Sodium: 163mg

Pesto Sauce

Prep time: 5 minutes / Serves: 16

VEGETARIAN, QUICK-PREP, UNDER 10 MINUTES

Pesto is a great sauce to have on hand for a variety of dishes, but certified low-FODMAP pesto sauce that does not contain garlic is hard to find. Making your own pesto is easy and delicious though. You can drizzle this multipurpose sauce over eggs or roasted vegetables, use it as a pizza sauce, mix with mayonnaise for a salad dressing, use as a sandwich spread, and so much more.

¾ **cup fresh basil leaves**

⅛ **cup Garlic-Infused Oil (page 134)**

¼ **cup pine nuts**

⅛ **cup extra-virgin olive oil**

⅛ **teaspoon sea salt**

⅛ **teaspoon freshly ground black pepper**

½ **cup freshly grated Parmesan cheese**

Combine the basil, oil, and pine nuts in a food processor and pulse until coarsely chopped. Add the olive oil, salt, pepper, and cheese and process until all are fully incorporated and smooth.

Storage tip: Store in an airtight container in the refrigerator for up to 1 week. Pesto freezes well and thaws quickly, so consider doubling the recipe to have extra to freeze. Freeze in ice cube trays, and then store the frozen pesto cubes in plastic freezer bags in the freezer for up to 6 months.

Per serving: Calories: 56; Total fat: 6g; Total carbs: 0g; Fiber: 0g; Sugar: 0g; Protein: 2g; Sodium: 33mg

Creamy Cilantro Taco Sauce

Prep time: 2 minutes / Serves: 10

NUT-FREE, QUICK-PREP, UNDER 10 MINUTES

If you're really into condiments and love dressing up your food, you will love this dreamy taco sauce. It goes smashingly well with the Easy Weeknight Fish Tacos (page 87). This sauce also tastes great as a sandwich condiment or spread on a low-FODMAP wrap.

½ **cup strained Greek yogurt**

¼ **cup fresh cilantro**

¼ **teaspoon ground cumin**

½ **tablespoon chopped scallions, green parts only**

1 **teaspoon lime juice**

⅛ **teaspoon kosher salt or more**

¼ **teaspoon freshly ground black pepper or more**

Combine the yogurt, cilantro, cumin, scallions, lime juice, salt, and pepper in a blender or food processor. Blend for 1 minute or until creamy.

Storage tip: Store in an airtight container in the refrigerator for 5 to 7 days.

Per serving: Calories: 15; Total fat: 0g; Total carbs: 1g; Fiber: 0g; Sugar: 1g; Protein: 1g; Sodium: 7mg

Chimichurri Sauce

Prep time: 10 minutes / Cook time: 5 minutes, plus 2 hours to chill / Serves: 12

NUT-FREE, VEGAN, UNDER 20 MINUTES

When I visited Argentina with my husband and family, I thoroughly remember the vibrant green chimichurri sauce served along with Argentina's famous beef. Traditional Argentinian chimichurri sauce contains high-FODMAP garlic and onion. This low-FODMAP version gets its garlic and onion flavor from asafetida powder and Garlic-Infused Oil (page 134). It's free of worry and can be used on beef, chicken, shellfish, and fish.

2 cups packed fresh Italian parsley

¼ cup packed fresh oregano leaves

1 tablespoon lime juice

¼ cup red wine vinegar

⅛ teaspoon asafetida powder

½ teaspoon red pepper flakes

½ teaspoon kosher salt

⅛ teaspoon freshly ground black pepper

¾ cup Garlic-Infused Oil (page 134)

1. Pulse the parsley and oregano in a food processor until finely chopped. Add the lime juice, vinegar, asafetida powder, red pepper flakes, salt, and pepper. Pulse again to combine. Turn the food processor on again and leave the motor running, then add the oil slowly. Scrape down the sides of the bowl and pulse a few more times until well combined.

2. Transfer the chimichurri sauce to an airtight container and refrigerate at least 2 hours before using. Refrigerate the sauce for up to 1 day before using to allow the flavors to become more potent.

3. Before serving, stir and season with more of the lime juice, asafetida powder, salt, or pepper if desired.

Ingredient tip: Dried oregano can be used for this sauce, but fresh oregano is better if your local grocer has it.

Preparation tip: When using asafetida powder for any recipe, take caution with how much you use as it is very potent. Try a little at a time to see how you like it.

Per serving: Calories: 118; Total fat: 13g; Total carbs: 2g; Fiber: 1g; Sugar: 0g; Protein: 1g; Sodium: 103mg

Teriyaki Sauce

Prep time: 5 minutes / Cook time: 10 minutes / Makes: 1¼ cups

NUT-FREE, VEGETARIAN, QUICK-PREP, UNDER 20 MINUTES

Forget the FODMAPs, this yummy Teriyaki Sauce doesn't contain garlic! Unless you make this recipe or use a certified low-FODMAP version, teriyaki sauce will always contain garlic or may contain large amounts of honey. This sticky-sweet recipe is safe to consume at 1 tablespoon per serving and so irresistible with chicken, pork, beef, salmon, in a stir-fry, or drizzled on bacon-wrapped scallops.

2 tablespoons cornstarch

1¼ cups cold water, divided

5 tablespoons packed brown sugar

⅛ teaspoon asafetida powder

1 teaspoon Garlic-Infused Oil (page 134)

¼ cup soy sauce

2 tablespoons honey

½ teaspoon ground ginger

1. In a small bowl, combine the cornstarch with ¼ cup of cold water and whisk until dissolved. Set aside.

2. In a medium saucepan set over medium heat, add the remaining 1 cup of water with the brown sugar, asafetida powder, oil, soy sauce, honey, and ginger. Stir to combine, then add the cornstarch mixture to the saucepan and stir to combine again.

3. Heat the sauce until it thickens, 7 to 10 minutes. If the sauce becomes too thick for your liking, add more water to thin it out. Use immediately.

Storage tip: Store in an airtight sterilized jar in the refrigerator for 2 to 3 weeks.

Per serving (2 tablespoons): Calories: 22; Total fat: 0g; Total carbs: 5g; Fiber: 0g; Sugar: 4g; Protein: 0g; Sodium: 181mg

Garlic-Infused Oil

Prep time: 5 minutes / Cook time: 5 minutes / Serves: 20

5 INGREDIENTS OR LESS, NUT-FREE, VEGAN, QUICK-PREP, UNDER 20 MINUTES

Garlic-Infused Oil is another one of my top low-FODMAP staples. When you miss the taste of garlic, this is a great and safe way to enjoy the taste without the fructans. Use this recipe lovingly on roasted vegetables, mashed potatoes, in dressings or marinades, for "garlic" bread, or in other recipes in this book.

6 medium garlic cloves, peeled and crushed

1¾ cups extra-virgin olive oil

1 to 1½ teaspoons red pepper flakes or another herb or spice (optional)

1. Peel the garlic and use a garlic press to crush the cloves.

2. Pour the olive oil into a small sauté pan and add the crushed garlic. Add your favorite herb or spice (if using). Cook over medium-low heat, stirring often, until the aromatics from the garlic release their fragrance, 3 to 5 minutes. The garlic should be just about crispy and light brown in color. Don't overcook; otherwise the oil will become bitter in taste.

3. Once ready, remove from the heat. Place a wire mesh strainer over a sanitized mason jar or container with an airtight lid and strain the oil. No pieces of garlic are to remain in the oil. Alternatively, you can forgo straining at first, and pour the garlic and oil into a container and allow it to sit for 1 to 2 hours before straining and removing the garlic pieces.

Ingredient tip: Try flavoring your garlic oil with ingredients like red pepper flakes, dried thyme, dried rosemary, dried basil, ground cumin, dried oregano, peppercorns, and more.

Storage tip: Store in an airtight container in the refrigerator for up to 3 days or in the freezer for up to 1 month. The oil will solidify in the refrigerator and freezer, so be sure to bring the oil to room temperature before using.

Safety tip: According to the North American Olive Oil Association, when making infused oil there is a risk of botulism (*Clostridium botulinum*), and it can live in oxygen-free environments. The fresh garlic can be contaminated with these spores. Fresh produce also contains water, which allows the bacteria to live and grow. To prevent bacteria from growing, be sure to sanitize your storage container beforehand, use dried herbs, and keep infused oils in the refrigerator for up to 3 days only.

Per serving: Calories: 153; Total fat: 18g; Total carbs: 0g; Fiber: 0g; Sugar: 0g; Protein: 0g; Sodium: 0mg

Shallot-Infused Oil

Prep time: 2 minutes / Cook time: 25 minutes / Serves: 24

5 INGREDIENTS OR LESS, NUT-FREE, VEGAN, QUICK-PREP, UNDER 30 MINUTES

You can still enjoy the delicate flavor of shallots without the FODMAPs. Shallot-Infused Oil is a great option to use in sauces, marinades, dressings, or as a dipping oil with low-FODMAP bread. Combine this oil with fresh rosemary and thyme to create a marinade for meat or use it in your next dressing recipe.

2 large shallots

1½ cups extra-virgin olive oil

1. Peel the shallots and rinse under running water, then pat dry. Slice them thinly on the cross section.

2. In a small sauté pan, heat the oil over medium-high and add 1 piece of shallot to the oil. Once it starts to sizzle, add the rest of the shallots and turn the heat down to medium. Fry the shallots until they turn from golden to brown, 8 to 10 minutes, then turn off the heat and move the pan off the burner. Keep the shallots in the oil and let them fry until they turn darker brown in color, 10 to 15 minutes.

3. Allow the oil to cool for a few minutes, then place a wire mesh strainer over a sanitized mason jar or container with an airtight lid and strain the oil. No pieces of shallots are to remain in the oil.

Safety Tip: According to the North American Olive Oil Association, when making infused oil there is a risk of botulism (*Clostridium botulinum*), and it can live in oxygen-free environments. The fresh shallots can be contaminated with these spores. Fresh produce also contains water, which allows the bacteria to live and grow. To prevent bacteria from growing, be sure to sanitize your storage container beforehand, use dried herbs, and keep infused oils in the refrigerator for up to 3 days only.

Per serving: Calories: 109; Total fat: 13g; Total carbs: 0g; Fiber: 0g; Sugar: 0g; Protein: 0g; Sodium: 0mg

Maple Vinaigrette

Prep time: 2 minutes / **Serves:** 12

NUT-FREE, VEGAN, QUICK-PREP, UNDER 10 MINUTES

This Maple Vinaigrette recipe is perfect with the Bacon Pecan Quinoa Salad (page 48). You can also try this dressing with your favorite combination of low-FODMAP greens, nuts, and cheese or in a low-FODMAP grain, nuts, and dried fruit salad (always watch servings of low-FODMAP dried fruits).

¼ cup extra-virgin olive oil

¼ cup maple syrup

2 tablespoons apple cider vinegar

1 tablespoon freshly squeezed lemon juice

¼ teaspoon kosher salt

⅛ teaspoon freshly ground black pepper

Add the olive oil, maple syrup, apple cider vinegar, lemon juice, salt, and pepper to a bowl and whisk until combined.

Storage tip: Store in an airtight container or mason jar in the refrigerator for up to 2 weeks.

Per serving: Calories: 54; Total fat: 4g; Total carbs: 5g; Fiber: 0g; Sugar: 4g; Protein: 0g; Sodium: 13mg

Carrot Ginger Dressing

Prep time: 10 minutes / Makes: 1⅓ cups

NUT-FREE, VEGETARIAN, UNDER 20 MINUTES

If you've ever had sushi at a Japanese restaurant, chances are you were served a green salad with a dressing like this Carrot Ginger Dressing. This low-FODMAP version is refreshing, bright, and delicious on just about any salad but also pairs perfectly with the Colorful Crunchy Salad (page 50). One to 2 tablespoons of this dressing is low-FODMAP.

⅓ cup extra-virgin olive oil

⅓ cup rice vinegar

2 large carrots, peeled and roughly chopped (about ⅔ cup)

1 tablespoon peeled and finely diced fresh ginger

2 tablespoons lime juice

1 tablespoon maple syrup

1 teaspoon honey

⅛ teaspoon kosher salt, plus more for seasoning

In a blender, combine the olive oil, vinegar, carrots, ginger, lime juice, maple syrup, honey, and salt. Blend until smooth. Taste, and add additional salt if desired, more maple syrup, or for more zing, add 1 to 2 teaspoons additional fresh ginger.

Ingredient tip: Honey is allowed on the low-FODMAP diet only at 1 teaspoon per serving. Clover honey is allowed only at ½ teaspoon per serving.

Per serving (2 tablespoons): Calories: 39; Total fat: 3g; Total carbs: 2g; Fiber: 0g; Sugar: 1g; Protein: 0g; Sodium: 9mg

Tahini Dressing

Prep time: 10 minutes / **Serves:** 12

NUT-FREE, VEGETARIAN, UNDER 20 MINUTES

Tahini Dressing will often call for high-FODMAPs such as garlic or honey. For this version, I've used Garlic-Infused Oil (page 134) and maple syrup, two low-FODMAP staples I use in the kitchen. Use this dressing in salads, Buddha bowls and quinoa bowls; drizzle it over roasted vegetables like roasted carrots (page 41), tofu dishes, sandwiches, and so much more.

Tahini

2 tablespoons freshly squeezed lemon juice

1 tablespoon maple syrup

1 tablespoon rice vinegar

½ tablespoon Garlic-Infused Oil (page 134) or toasted sesame oil

⅛ teaspoon sea salt

⅛ teaspoon freshly ground black pepper

2 tablespoons water

1. Into a small bowl, scoop out ¼ cup of tahini, taking care to get as much of the paste as possible, leaving the oil in the jar.

2. Add the lemon juice, maple syrup, rice vinegar, oil, sea salt, and pepper, whisking until well combined. Whisk in the water 2 teaspoons at a time until smooth. Add more lemon juice, maple syrup, salt, or pepper to taste. Store in a mason jar or other jar with a tight-fitting lid.

Storage tip: This dressing will keep well in the refrigerator in an airtight container for about 1 week. If the dressing thickens, simply thin it with a little water as needed.

Per serving: Calories: 41; Total fat: 3g; Total carbs: 2g; Fiber: 1g; Sugar: 1g; Protein: 1g; Sodium: 26mg

Sweet and Spicy Dressing

Prep time: 2 minutes / Makes: ¼ cup

NUT-FREE, VEGAN, QUICK-PREP, UNDER 10 MINUTES

You'll love how the sweetness from the maple syrup and rice wine vinegar mixes with the spiciness of the sriracha and adds a kick to an otherwise bland or unexciting salad. Enliven your next green salad with this dressing, your choice of protein, 1 tablespoon of slivered almonds, 1 ounce of goat cheese, and ¼ cup of blueberries (per serving). This dressing also tastes delicious over grilled pineapple.

¼ **teaspoon kosher salt**

⅛ **teaspoon freshly ground black pepper**

3 **tablespoons Garlic-Infused Oil (page 134)**

1 **tablespoon maple syrup**

2 **tablespoons rice wine vinegar**

3 **teaspoons sriracha**

In a small mason jar, combine the salt, pepper, oil, maple syrup, and vinegar. Secure the lid on the jar and shake well. Add the sriracha 1 teaspoon at a time until the desired heat level is achieved, shaking the jar well between additions.

Storage tip: Store leftover dressing in the refrigerator for up to 14 days. Bring to room temperature and shake well before each use.

Per serving (2 tablespoons): Calories: 111; Total fat: 11g; Total carbs: 4g; Fiber: 0g; Sugar: 4g; Protein: 0g; Sodium: 86mg

Strawberry Salad Dressing

Prep time: 2 minutes / Serves: 4

DAIRY-FREE, NUT-FREE, VEGAN OPTION, QUICK-PREP, UNDER 10 MINUTES

Strawberry spinach salad is one of my favorite low-FODMAP salads. It's so easy to whip up and is super healthy, too. Use this dressing in a salad with strawberries, baby spinach, feta or goat cheese, walnuts, and a low-FODMAP serving of avocado. It's also delicious in quinoa salads or over a low-FODMAP berry salad.

½ **tablespoon poppy seeds**

½ **cup granulated sugar**

½ **cup Shallot-Infused Oil (page 136)**

¼ **cup rice wine vinegar**

¼ **teaspoon paprika**

¼ **teaspoon Worcestershire sauce (for the vegan option, see FODMAP tip on page 68)**

In a medium bowl, whisk together the poppy seeds, sugar, oil, vinegar, paprika, and Worcestershire sauce. Cover and chill for 1 hour before using on salad.

Storage tip: Store in a mason jar or an airtight container in the refrigerator for up to 2 weeks. If the oil in the dressing has hardened from refrigeration, allow the dressing to sit until the oil has melted, and whisk before serving.

Per serving: Calories: 326; Total fat: 26g; Total carbs: 25g; Fiber: 0g; Sugar: 25g; Protein: 0g; Sodium: 4mg

Asian-Style Salad Dressing

Prep time: 5 minutes / Makes: ½ cup

DAIRY-FREE, NUT-FREE, VEGETARIAN, QUICK-PREP, UNDER 10 MINUTES

This dressing pairs well with my Crunchy Asian-Inspired Salad (page 45) and also tastes lovely over a low-FODMAP salad of romaine, carrots, and other crunchy low-FODMAP vegetables served with marinated salmon, grilled shrimp, or grilled tofu.

3 tablespoons sesame oil

3 tablespoons rice vinegar

2 teaspoons honey

1½ tablespoons brown sugar

1 tablespoon fresh lime juice

2 teaspoons freshly grated ginger

⅛ teaspoon kosher salt

⅛ teaspoon freshly ground black pepper

In a medium bowl or mason jar, whisk together the oil, vinegar, honey, brown sugar, lime juice, ginger, salt, and pepper.

Ingredient tip: One teaspoon of honey is equal to one low-FODMAP serving.

Storage tip: Store in an airtight container in the refrigerator for up to 1 week.

Per serving (2 tablespoons): Calories: 64; Total fat: 5g; Total carbs: 4g; Fiber: 0g; Sugar: 3g; Protein: 0g; Sodium: 36mg

Flax Egg (Egg Replacer)

Prep time: 2 minutes, plus 5 minutes to sit / Serves: 1

5 INGREDIENTS OR LESS, NUT-FREE, VEGAN, QUICK-PREP, UNDER 10 MINUTES

Flaxseeds and water create a gelatinous texture, which allows them to function similarly to eggs. Flax eggs are great for anyone watching their cholesterol, and they're a great source of fiber and the omega-3 fatty acids. Use a Flax Egg in denser recipes such as cookies, brownies, muffins, or pancakes. This recipe replaces exactly one egg.

1 tablespoon ground flaxseeds

2½ tablespoons filtered water (room temperature is best)

1. Put the flaxseeds in a blender and pulse until finely ground.

2. Combine the flaxseeds and water in a bowl. Stir to combine. Allow to sit for 5 minutes to set before using in a recipe. Double or triple the amounts as needed.

Ingredient tip: Other vegan "egg" substitutes include ¼ cup of mashed sweet potato, a mashed half of a (firm) banana, and 1 tablespoon of ground chia seeds mixed with 3 tablespoons of hot water.

Per serving: Calories: 46; Total fat: 3g; Total carbs: 3g; Fiber: 2g; Sugar: 1g; Protein: 2g; Sodium: 3mg

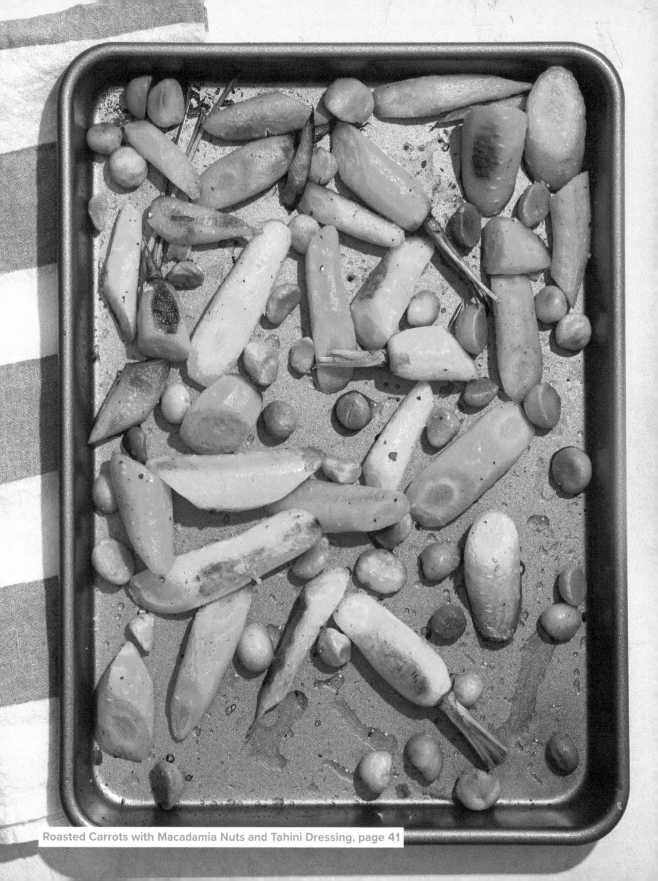

Roasted Carrots with Macadamia Nuts and Tahini Dressing, page 41

Low-FODMAP Foods

Barbeque Sauce (Fody™ Low FODMAP)
Black and/or green olives
Capers, salted or in vinegar
Canned tomatoes (without onion or garlic)
Fish sauce
Horseradish
Jam, marmalade
Jam, strawberry
Ketchup (certified low-FODMAP such as Fody™)
Mayonnaise
Mint sauce
Oyster sauce

Pasta sauce (certified low-FODMAP such as Prego® Sensitive Recipe
Peanut butter
Polenta
Soy sauce
Sriracha, 1 teaspoon
Stevia powder (such as Pyure® Organic Stevia)
Sweet and sour sauce
Tomato paste
Vinegar—Apple cider, Balsamic (1 tablespoon), Red wine, Rice wine
Worcestershire sauce, 2 tablespoons

Herbs and Spices

Asafoetida powder
Basil
Bay leaves
Cardamom
Chilli powder
Cilantro
Cinnamon
Cloves
Coriander, seeds and fresh
Cumin
Curry leaves, fresh
Curry powder
Dill
Fennel seeds
Fenugreek leaves, dried; seeds
Five spice
Goraka
Gotukala
Kaffir lime leaves
Lemongrass

Mint
Mustard seeds
Mustard, yellow or Dijon
Nutmeg
Oregano
Pandan leaves
Parsley
Pepper, black
Rampa leaves
Rosemary
Saffron
Sage
Star anise
Tarragon
Thai basil
Thyme
Turmeric
Vanilla
Wasabi, paste, powder
Watercress

Vegetables

Arugula
Bean sprouts
*Bell pepper, green
Bell pepper, red
*Broccoli
*Butternut squash
*Cabbage, common (green)
*Cabbage, red
Carrot
Collard greens
Corn, baby, canned
Cucumber
Eggplant/Aubergine
*Fennel, bulb and leaves
Ginger
Jalapeño
Kale
*Leek, leaves
Lettuce, butter, iceberg, red, romaine

Mushrooms, champignons, canned
Olives, black, green
Onion, spring, scallion, green tips only
Parsnip
Potato, unpeeled
*Potato, sweet
Radish
Rutbagas
Seaweed (nori)
*Spinach, baby
Squash, pattypan
Swiss chard
Tomato, canned
*Tomato, cherry
*Tomato, Roma
*Turnip
Water chestnuts
*Zucchini

Fruits

Acai powder
Banana, firm
*Blueberries
Breadfruit
*Cantaloupe
Carambola
Clementine
*Coconut
*Cranberries, dried
Dragon fruit
*Goji berries, dried
Grapes (all)

Guava, ripe
*Kiwi
Orange, navel
Papaya (yellow)
*Passionfruit
Plantain
*Raisins
Rhubarb
Strawberries
Tamarind

Dairy

Butter

Cheese

- Brie
- Camembert
- Cheddar
- Colby
- Feta
- Havarti
- Mozzarella
- Pecorino
- Swiss

Ghee

Lactose-free kefir

Milk

- Lactose-free
- Macadamia
- Quinoa, unsweetened
- Rice
- Soy (made from soy protein)
- Almond

Yogurt

- Almond
- Coconut
- Lactose-free (made with low-FODMAP fruit, no honey, inulin, high-fructose corn syrup or other high-FODMAP ingredients)

Proteins

Bacon

Beef

Canned salmon (in brine)

Canned sardines (canned in oil)

Canned tuna (canned in brine or oil)

Chicken

Eggs

Fish

Lamb

Pork

Shellfish

Tempeh

Tofu (only firm, not silken)

Turkey

*All of the above are low-FODMAP as long as not marinated or processed with high-FODMAP ingredients

Grains, Pastas, Seeds, Flours

Bran, oat or rice

Bread (with no added high-FODMAPs)

Buckwheat

Corn

Corn flakes

Couscous, gluten-free, made with maize flour

Gluten-free (no high FODMAP ingredients e.g., inulin, besan flour)

Millet

Spelt, 100% spelt, sourdough

Spelt, sourdough

Wheat, white, sourdough

Wheat, wholemeal, sourdough

Arrowroot flour

Buckwheat flour

Corn flour

Gluten-free pasta (no high FODMAP ingredients e.g., legume flours, inulin)

Gluten-free, plain flour

Kelp noodles

Maize flour

Millet

Millet flour

Oats

Quinoa

Quinoa flour

Rice

Rice flakes

Rice flour, plain or roasted

Rice noodles

Sorghum flour

Spelt flour

Teff

Teff flour

Vermicelli noodles

Wheat pasta (½ cup serve or less)

Yam flour

Nuts and Seeds

Brazil nuts

Peanuts

Quinoa

Sunflower seeds

Walnuts

Fats and Oils

Canola oil

Extra-virgin olive oil

Garlic-infused oil

Shallot-infused oil

Sweeteners

Cane sugar

**Golden syrup ½ tablespoon per serving

**Honey (only at 1 teaspoon per serving)

Maple syrup

Table sugar

Beverages

Coffee

**Coconut water (½ cup)

Cranberry juice

Tea

**Indicates this food can become moderate to high in FODMAPs. Always follow suggested servings. Alternatively if you are using a food that could potentially become moderate to high in FODMAPs and you are not sure about the weight or volume, you can always use an electronic food scale.

The Dirty Dozen and the Clean Fifteen™

A nonprofit environmental watchdog organization called Environmental Working Group (EWG) looks at data supplied by the US Department of Agriculture (USDA) and the Food and Drug Administration (FDA) about pesticide residues. Each year it compiles a list of the best and worst pesticide loads found in commercial crops. You can use these lists to decide which fruits and vegetables to buy organic to minimize your exposure to pesticides and which produce is considered safe enough to buy conventionally. This does not mean they are pesticide-free, though, so wash these fruits and vegetables thoroughly. The list is updated annually, and you can find it online at EWG.org/FoodNews.

Dirty Dozen™

1. strawberries
2. spinach
3. kale
4. nectarines
5. apples
6. grapes
7. peaches
8. cherries
9. pears
10. tomatoes
11. celery
12. potatoes

†Additionally, nearly three-quarters of hot pepper samples contained pesticide residues.

Clean Fifteen™

1. avocados
2. sweet corn
3. pineapples
4. sweet peas (frozen)
5. onions
6. papayas
7. eggplants
8. asparagus
9. kiwis
10. cabbages
11. cauliflower
12. cantaloupes
13. broccoli
14. mushrooms
15. honeydew melons

Measurement Conversions

Volume Equivalents (Liquid)

US STANDARD	US STANDARD (OUNCES)	METRIC (APPROXIMATE)
2 tablespoons	1 fl. oz.	30 mL
¼ cup	2 fl. oz.	60 mL
½ cup	4 fl. oz.	120 mL
1 cup	8 fl. oz.	240 mL
1 ½ cups	12 fl. oz.	355 mL
2 cups or 1 pint	16 fl. oz.	475 mL
4 cups or 1 quart	32 fl. oz.	1 L
1 gallon	128 fl. oz.	4 L

Oven Temperatures

FAHRENHEIT	CELSIUS (APPROXIMATE)
250°F	120°C
300°F	150°C
325°F	165°C
350°F	180°C
375°F	190°C
400°F	200°C
425°F	220°C
450°F	230°C

Volume Equivalents (Dry)

US STANDARD	METRIC (APPROXIMATE)
⅛ teaspoon	0.5 mL
¼ teaspoon	1 mL
½ teaspoon	2 mL
¾ teaspoon	4 mL
1 teaspoon	5 mL
1 tablespoon	15 mL
¼ cup	59 mL
⅓ cup	79 mL
½ cup	118 mL
⅔ cup	156 mL
¾ cup	177 mL
1 cup	235 mL
2 cups or 1 pint	475 mL
3 cups	700 mL
4 cups or 1 quart	1 L

Weight Equivalents

US STANDARD	METRIC (APPROXIMATE)
½ ounce	15 g
1 ounce	30 g
2 ounces	60 g
4 ounces	115 g
8 ounces	225 g
12 ounces	340 g
16 ounces or 1 pound	455 g

Resources

Websites

bit.ly/FODMAPCourse

Head over to **bit.ly/FODMAPCourse (https://fodmap-life.teachable.com/p/low-fodmap -diet-beginners-course)** to learn more about The Low-FODMAP Diet Beginner's Course. This course has all the information you need for the diet in one place, with tips and guidance from registered dietitians.

Everydaynutrition.com.au

As registered and Accredited Practicing Dietitians in Melbourne, Joanna Baker, APD, AN, RN, and Marnie Nitschke APD, AN, are experts in the relationship between diet and disease and are able to provide professional evidence-based advice to complement medical intervention and support patients in identifying and managing their individual condition. They focus on translating the very latest in gut health research into real food terms, providing practical everyday strategies so that you can eat well, be well, and feel great.

FODMAPLife.com

For everything low-FODMAP, head over to Colleen Francioli's website, FODMAPLife.com where you will find low-FODMAP recipes, eBooks, handouts, meal plans, tips, resources, news, and more.

FODMAP Friendly Program Certified Products—fodmapfriendly.com/certified-products

Katescarlata.com

Kate Scarlata is a Boston-based registered and licensed dietitian, and a *New York Times* bestselling author with 25+ years of experience. She is a world-renowned low-FODMAP diet expert and invited speaker at numerous international and national gastrointestinal health conferences from Harvard Medical School to Monash University.

Monash University Low-FODMAP Certified™—www.monashfodmap.com/product -and-recipe-certification-program/our-certified-partners

Apps

FODMAP Friendly App | **FODMAP Friendly**—fodmapfriendly.com/app

The Monash University FODMAP App—www.monashfodmap.com/ibs-central /i-have-ibs/get-the-app/

Books

The Bloated Belly Whisperer: See Results Within a Week and Tame Digestive Distress Once and for All by Tamara Duker Freuman, MS, RD, CDN. St. Martin's Press, December 24, 2018. This book is the first evidence-based guide to understanding and treating the many different ways your belly can get bloated. Learn what causes bloating and how to avoid distressing digestive symptoms.

The Complete Low-FODMAP Diet: A Revolutionary Plan for Managing IBS and Other Digestive Disorders by Sue Shepherd and Peter Gibson. The Experiment, August 13, 2013. This excellent book is the first of its kind and is a "classic." It is authored by Sue Shepherd and Peter Gibson, who were part of the team that created the low-FODMAP diet. Though the book is only six years old, some of the information in the book is outdated because the low-FODMAP diet has evolved much over the years.

Digestive Health With REAL Food, **2nd Edition, Updated and Expanded** by Aglaee Jacob. Paleo Media, April 1, 2018. The first couple of chapters of this book make it easy to understand the human digestive system, basic functioning of a healthy digestive system, and how digestion can go wrong.

The Low-FODMAP Diet for Beginners: A 7-Day Plan to Beat Bloat and Soothe Your Gut with Recipes for Fast IBS Relief by Mollie Tunitsky and Gabriela Gardner, RDN-AP LD CNSC. Rockridge Press, October 10, 2017. This book makes it simple and accessible to discover relief from IBS and upset guts.

The Low-FODMAP Diet Step by Step: A Personalized Plan to Relieve the Symptoms of IBS and Other Digestive Disorders—with More Than 130 Deliciously Satisfying Recipes by Kate Scarlata and Dédé Wilson. Da Capo Lifelong Books. December 19, 2017. One of the more up-to-date books on the low-FODMAP diet with expertise from registered dietitian and FODMAP expert Kate Scarlata and featuring delicious recipes from Dédé Wilson, co-founder of FODMAP Everyday.

Organizations

Academy of Nutrition and Dietetics—www.eatright.org

American Gastroenterological Association—https://www.gastro.org/

GI Society, Canadian Society of Intestinal Research—https://badgut.org

IFFGD, the International Foundation for Functional Gastrointestinal Disorders—https://www.aboutibs.org

Groups

Facebook has many private groups focusing on the low-FODMAP diet. These groups are great places to meet others following the diet, to ask your questions, and best of all, to get support. Here are a few that you may consider joining:

- FODMAP Life Support Group
- FODMAP UK
- Irritable Bowel Syndrome IBS Support
- Low FODMAP Australia
- Low FODMAP Diet Support
- Low FODMAP Recipes and Support

Brands

The following represents a list of certified low-FODMAP products that you can find at your local grocery store or online. For more products available in the United States, Australia, New Zealand, the United Kingdom, and Canada, please visit the Monash FODMAP and FODMAP friendly websites:

Campbell Soup Company®—Prego® Sensitive Recipe (pasta sauce)

Casa de Sante™—salsa, pasta sauce, stock powder, rubs, teas, snack bars, and more

Enjoy Life®—various snacks and chocolate

FODMAPPED Foods—soups, simmer sauces, pasta sauces, ready-made meals, and more

Fody Foods™—garlic-infused oil, condiments, dressings, marinades, potato chips, snack bars, and more

FreshCap Mushrooms—THRIVE 6 all natural mushroom extract blend and ELECTRIC 100% pure Lion's Mane Mushroom Extract

Green Valley Creamery—lactose-free yogurt, kefir, cream cheese, and sour cream

Kellogg's®—gluten-free Special K and Corn Flakes

LAIKI—rice crackers

Live Free Foods—salad dressings

Three Arrows—collagen peptides

TrueSelf—snack bars

*If your local grocer does not carry these products, you can always ask the manager to special order products for you! You can also ask them to test out selling the products in the store—others with IBS in your community need low-FODMAP products, just like you.

References

Barrett J. S., Gearry R. B., Muir J. G., Irving P. M., Rose R, Rosella O, Haines M. L., Shepherd S. J., Gibson, P. R. (April 2010). "Dietary Poorly Absorbed, Short-Chain Carbohydrates Increase Delivery of Water and Fermentable Substrates to the Proximal Colon." *Alimentary Pharmacology & Therapeutics.*

Gibson P. R. (March 2017). "History of the Low FODMAP Diet." *Journal of Gastroenterology and Hepatology (Review).*

Gibson P. R., Shepherd S. J. (June 2005). "Personal View: Food for Thought—Western Lifestyle and Susceptibility to Crohn's Disease. The FODMAP Hypothesis." *Alimentary Pharmacology & Therapeutics.*

Hill, P., Muir, J. G. PhD, and Gibson P. R. (January 13, 2017). "Controversies and Recent Developments of the Low-FODMAP Diet Gastroenterology and Hepatology." *The Independent Peer-Reviewed Journal*, US National Library of Medicine, National Institutes of Health.

Nanayakkara, W. S., Skidmore P. M., ML, O'Brien L., Wilkinson T. J., and Gearry, R. B. (June 17, 2016). "Efficacy of the Low FODMAP Diet for Treating Irritable Bowel Syndrome: The Evidence to Date."

Staudacher H. M., Whelan, K. (2017) "The Low FODMAP Diet: Recent Advances in Understanding Its Mechanisms and Efficacy in IBS." *BMJ Journals, Gut.*

Varney J. & Tuck, C. (November 16, 2017). "Enzyme Therapy can Help Reduce Symptoms in IBS Patients Sensitive to Galacto-Oligosaccharides (GOS)." Monash University FODMAP blog.

FODMAP Friendly App | FODMAP Friendly—fodmapfriendly.com/app

Food Sources of Lactose (PDF)—Dietitians of Canada

The history of Spaghetti alla puttanesca—Wikipedia

Monash University FODMAP Diet App—www.monashfodmap.com/ibs-central/i-have
-ibs/get-the-app/

Read this before making homemade infused olive oil: The North American Olive Oil
Association February 21, 2017. https://www.aboutoliveoil.org/read-this-before
-making-homemade-infused-olive-oil

Reid, D.—www.theglobaldietitian.com

Rome IV Diagnostic Criteria for Irritable Bowel Syndrome (IBS)—MD+CALC
https://www.mdcalc.com/rome-iv-diagnostic-criteria-irritable-bowel-syndrome
-ibs#pearls-pitfalls

What are Functional Bowel Disorders (FBD)?—University of Michigan, Michigan Medicine. https://www.med.umich.edu/fbd/

Index

Acknowledgments

I would like to thank the following people:

Joanna Baker APD, AN, RN, everydaynutrition.com.au, for working on this book, thoroughly reviewing it, and providing the necessary expertise needed to safely guide readers along through every chapter. Learning about the low-FODMAP diet can be difficult, but Joanna's warm approach to education and to people is greatly appreciated by many across the world.

Diana Reid, MPH, RD, theglobaldietitian.com, her guidance has gone beyond the low-FODMAP diet and has been invaluable to me as an educator in nutrition and wellness. I highly respect her passion for her work and the level of caring she gives to people with IBS.

Kate Scarlata, RDN, LDN, katescarlata.com, for her guidance and help over the years, and for being a wonderful inspiration in her caring and fun approach to teaching others about the low-FODMAP diet. Her expertise and hard work (along with help from her daughter Chelsea) has greatly helped to spread the word about FODMAPs, IBS, and gut health.

Mimi Clark, vegan chef and pioneer in plant-based cooking, veggourmet.wordpress.com—for her sweet friendship and guidance, and for always pushing me to be my best.

Hannah Kaminsky, food writer and photographer of MySweetVegan.com, for her knowledge with vegan cuisine and her innovative, absolutely delicious, and flavorful ideas.

And finally, thank you to Callisto Media for inviting me to do this book. It has been a pleasure working with the team and collaborating on ideas.

About the Author

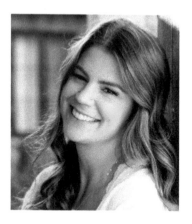

Colleen Francioli, CNC is the founder of FODMAP Life. She is a certified nutritionist, an author of two cookbooks, and a marketing consultant. Colleen once suffered from IBS herself and has since found life balance with the low-FODMAP diet. Colleen started FODMAPLife.com to help others with IBS learn how to choose the right foods and make stress relief a priority for a balanced mind-body approach to gut health.

Colleen has her own online school called The Low-FODMAP Diet Beginner's Course and features the expertise of FODMAP-trained dietitians to provide only the best and most sound advice and guidance for the diet. She has been featured on *The Intolerant Cooks* show in Australia, in commercials, and on podcasts and has given talks about the low-FODMAP diet. As a marketing consultant, she's represented different health and wellness brands and is a regular at the Natural Products Expo West, where she enjoys meeting new brands and trying new products. She is currently developing her own product line for the low-FODMAP diet.

Colleen leads an active life with her husband, Jeremy, and her sons Enzo and Luca. She lives in Colorado.

CPSIA information can be obtained
at www.ICGtesting.com
Printed in the USA
JSHW050949031121
19985JS00002B/2

9 781641 527194